LYMPHATIC DIET COOKBOOK FOR BEGINNERS

Wholesome Nutrition Strategies and Delicious Recipes to Nourish and Support Your Body's Natural Detox Pathways

Dr. Kelly Haaland

To show our appreciation for your purchase, we're delighted to offer you these special bonuses as a heartfelt thank you.

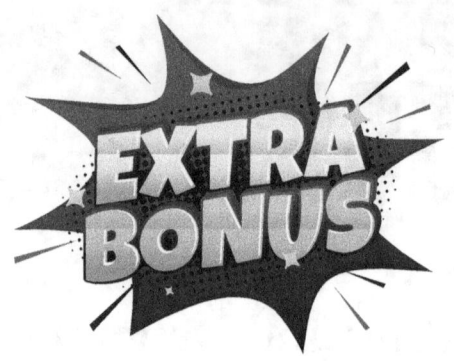 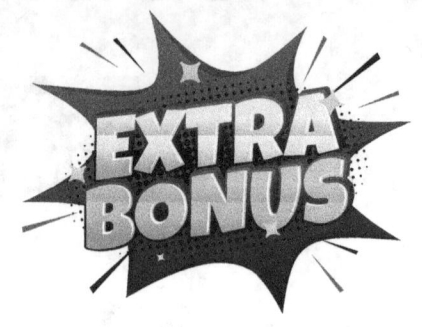

1. A Food Tracker Journal
2. Downloadable E-BOOK featuring full-color images of finished recipes
3. One-on-one consultation session with Dr. Kelly Haaland

Copyright © 2024 All rights reserved.

No part of this book may be reproduced or transmitted in any form or by any means, electronic or mechanical, including photocopying, recording, or by any information storage and retrieval system, without written permission from the author. The scanning, uploading, and distribution of this book via the internet or via any other means without the permission of the author is illegal and punishable by law. The author has made every effort to ensure the accuracy of the information contained in this book. However, the author cannot be held responsible for any errors or omissions.

TABLE OF CONTENTS

Chapter 1: Understanding the Lymphatic System
- Basics of the Lymphatic System..................................8
- Functions of the Lymphatic System..........................10

Chapter 2: Principles of the Lymphatic Diet
- Key Components of a Lymphatic Diet.........................12.
- Foods to Embrace...14
- Foods to Avoid...16

Brekfast Recipes
Coconut Chia Pudding..18
Tofu Scramble..19
Greek Yogurt with Nuts and Seeds................................20
Almond Butter Banana Wrap..21
Beetroot Smoothie...22
Cinnamon Apple Oatmeal..23
Breakfast Tacos...24
Zucchini Fritters..25
Acai Bowl..26
Spinach and Feta Crustless Quiche..............................27
Fruit Salad..28
Cauliflower Hash Browns..29
Lentil Porridge..30
Veggie Breakfast Burrito...31
Sweet Potato Toast...32
Buckwheat Pancakes..33
Coconut Yogurt Parfait..34
Vegetable Omelette..35
Berry Smoothie...36
Turmeric Scrambled Eggs...37
Green Smoothie Bowl...38

Vegetables Recipes
Grilled Asparagus with Lemon Zest............................39
Korean Spinach Side Dish..40

Swiss Chard Rolls......41
Szechuan Green Beans......42
Cabbage Stir-Fry......43
Spinach and Feta Stuffed Portobello Mushrooms......44
Mediterranean Roasted Vegetables......45
Okonomiyaki......46
Vietnamese Summer Rolls......47
Ratatouille Tian......48
Sesame Ginger Snap Peas......49
Stuffed Mushrooms......50
Vegetable Paella......51
Zucchini Noodles with Pesto......52
Thai Green Papaya Salad......53
Miso Glazed Eggplant......54
Italian Marinated Grilled Vegetables......55
Vegetable Spring Rolls......56
Cucumber Salad......57
Vegetable Curry......58
Caprese Salad......60
Greek Salad......61
Stuffed Bell Peppers......62

Poultry & Meat Recipes
American BBQ Chicken Drumsticks......63
German Sauerbraten......64
Thai Basil Beef......66
Mexican Chicken Tinga Tacos......67
Japanese Yakitori Skewers......68
Brazilian Feijoada......69
Swedish Meatballs......70
Lebanese Grilled Chicken Shawarma......71
Asian Orange Glazed Duck Breast......72
Italian Sausage and Kale Soup......74
Thai Green Curry Beef......75
Spanish Chicken and Chorizo Paella......76
Barbecue Pulled Pork......78
Indian Butter Chicken (Murgh Makhani)......79
French Coq au Vin......81
Chipotle Lime Grilled Shrimp......83

Sesame Ginger Turkey Stir-Fry..84
Greek Lemon Garlic Lamb Chops..85
Honey Mustard Glazed Salmon...86
Italian Meatballs..87
Vietnamese Lemongrass Chicken...88
Herb-Roasted Cornish Hens..89
Thai Basil Chicken..90

Fish & Seafood Recipes
Japanese Chirashi Sushi...91
Italian Cioppino..92
Thai Green Curry Mussels...93
American Grilled Halibut with Lemon and Herbs.................................94
Greek Grilled Shrimp Souvlaki...95
Japanese Sushi Nigiri...96
Italian Baked Cod with Cherry Tomatoes and Olives...........................97
Thai Fish Cakes (Tod Mun Pla)...98
Spanish Garlic Butter Shrimp...99
Japanese Grilled Miso Glazed Salmon...100
French Trout Almondine..101
Thai Coconut Lime Shrimp Soup...102
Italian Seafood Risotto...103
Vietnamese Shrimp Summer Rolls..105
Greek Grilled Swordfish...106
Japanese Teriyaki Glazed Salmon...107
American New England Clam Chowder...108
Spanish Seafood Paella...109
Thai Spicy Basil Squid (Pad Kra Pao Pla Meuk)...................................111
Italian Linguine with Clams..112
French Bouillabaisse...113
Thai Coconut Curry Shrimp...114

8-WEEK MEAL PLAN..115

BONUSES..125

Dear Esteemed Reader

As you turn each page, eager to explore and experiment with the wholesome recipes curated for your lymphatic health, we kindly remind you of the uniqueness of your body's narrative. Just as every individual has their own story, so too do our dietary needs differ, painted with the broad strokes of our personal health backgrounds, preferences, and nutritional requirements. It is with this understanding that we encourage you to approach these recipes not as rigid prescriptions, but as starting points for your culinary creativity and nutritional journey.

We advocate for a mindful adaptation of the recipes in this cookbook to suit your personal dietary needs. Should a particular ingredient not sit well with you, or if you find yourself puzzled by which choices will best align with your health goals, consider this an opportunity to tailor these dishes to your liking, ensuring they nourish you in the most beneficial way. In these moments of uncertainty, seeking the guidance of a healthcare professional or a registered dietitian can provide clarity and reassurance, ensuring that the path you choose supports your overall well-being.

Moreover, we acknowledge the fluid nature of nutritional information, which serves as a gentle reminder that the nutritional values provided alongside our recipes are approximate estimates. Variations in ingredient sizes, brands, and even the soil in which our foods are grown can influence these figures. As you embrace the practice of mindful eating, let this awareness encourage flexibility and an openness to adjustment, ensuring that your meals are not only delicious but also harmoniously aligned with your body's needs.

Moreover, If our cookbook has brought joy to your kitchen and table, we'd be thrilled to hear about your experiences in an Amazon review. On the flip side, if you stumble upon any hiccups while exploring our recipes, don't hesitate to get in touch at **kellyhaaland2@gmail.com** We're here to support your cooking journey every step of the way.

Introduction

Welcome to the "Lymphatic Diet Cookbook for Beginners," your gateway to a transformative journey that intertwines the art of cooking with the science of nurturing one of the most vital yet often overlooked systems in your body - the lymphatic system. This book is not just a list of recipes; it is a friend, a guide, and a companion for you as you set out to understand the deep influence that nutrition has on your health.

Imagine for a moment your body as an intricate city, bustling with activity, life, and energy. In this city, the lymphatic system functions like the unsung sanitation crew, tirelessly working behind the scenes to clean up, detoxify, and protect. It's a network of vessels and nodes that are pivotal in managing the fluid balance in your body, filtering out toxins, and supporting your immune system. Despite its crucial role, it's a system that doesn't often get the limelight it deserves, until now. This book is crafted for you, the beginner, with love and care, to gently guide you into the world of lymphatic health through the joy of cooking. It's for those who are curious, those who seek not only to eat but to nourish and flourish. Whether you're looking to support your lymphatic health due to a specific health condition or you're simply intrigued by the potential for enhanced energy and vitality, you're in the right place. As you flip through these pages, you'll find recipes that are as delicious as they are beneficial, designed to be approachable for cooks of all levels. But this cookbook aims to be more than just a collection of dishes; it's a treasure trove of knowledge, offering insights into how food can be your ally in maintaining and improving your lymphatic health.

We set out on this adventure with the understanding that your route to wellness is as individual as you are. Each body responds differently to food, and what nourishes one person may not have the same effect on another. This is why we encourage you to use this cookbook not as a strict rulebook, but as a source of inspiration. Feel empowered to tweak, modify, and experiment with the recipes to suit your taste buds and nutritional needs.

And remember, when in doubt, consulting with a healthcare provider can offer personalized guidance tailored to your health journey. Moreover, as you begin to integrate these meals into your daily life, remember that the nutritional values provided are estimates. Factors such as ingredient quality, preparation methods, and portion sizes can influence these numbers. We invite you to embrace this flexibility, allowing room for intuition and personal preference to guide your cooking experience.

So, dear reader, as you stand at the threshold of this exciting adventure, we invite you to step into the kitchen with an open heart and a curious mind. Let the **"Lymphatic Diet Cookbook for Beginners"** be your guide to exploring how the simple act of cooking and eating can be transformed into an act of self-care and love. Here's to your health, to your joy, and to a journey that's about to unfold deliciously before you. Welcome aboard!

Chapter 1: Understanding the Lymphatic System

What is the Lymphatic System?
The lymphatic system is a crucial part of the body's immune system. It's a network of vessels and organs that helps the body to rid itself of toxins, waste, and other unwanted materials. The primary function of the lymphatic system is to transport lymph, a clear fluid containing white blood cells, throughout the body. Lymph plays a vital role in immune function, as it helps to remove harmful substances from tissues and aids in the fight against infections.

Components of the Lymphatic System:
1. **Lymphatic Vessels:** These are a network of thin tubes that carry lymph fluid throughout the body. They resemble blood vessels but are smaller and have a one-way flow system.
2. **Lymph Nodes:** These are small, bean-shaped structures that filter lymph fluid and contain immune cells called lymphocytes, which help to fight infections. Lymph nodes are found throughout the body, with clusters in areas like the neck, armpits, and groin.
3. **Lymphatic Organs:** These include the spleen, thymus, and tonsils. These organs are involved in immune function and the production of white blood cells.
4. **Bone Marrow:** Bone marrow is responsible for producing lymphocytes, which are essential for the body's immune response.

Importance of a Healthy Lymphatic System:
A well-functioning lymphatic system is essential for overall health and well-being. It helps to support the body's immune function, maintain fluid balance, and promote proper digestion and nutrient absorption. When the lymphatic system becomes compromised or inefficient, it can lead to issues such as lymphedema (swelling due to fluid buildup), impaired immune function, and increased susceptibility to infections.

Hence, the lymphatic system is a critical component of the body's immune defense and overall health. Understanding its basics can help individuals take steps to support and maintain a healthy lymphatic system through lifestyle choices, including diet and exercise.

Functions of the Lymphatic System

1. **Immune Response:**
   - **Pathogen Defense:** The lymphatic system plays a vital role in defending the body against pathogens such as bacteria, viruses, and fungi. Lymph nodes, containing specialized immune cells like lymphocytes and macrophages, filter lymph fluid, trapping and destroying harmful substances.
   - **Antigen Presentation:** Lymph nodes serve as sites for antigen presentation, where immune cells display antigens (foreign substances) to activate other immune cells, initiating an immune response.
2. **Fluid Balance:**
   - **Lymphatic Drainage:** Lymphatic vessels collect excess fluid, proteins, and waste products from tissues and return them to the bloodstream. This prevents the buildup of fluid in tissues, maintaining fluid balance and preventing swelling (edema).
   - **Prevention of Edema:** By removing excess fluid, the lymphatic system helps prevent edema, a condition characterized by swelling due to fluid retention.
3. **Absorption of Dietary Fats and Fat-Soluble Vitamins:**
   - **Lacteals:** Specialized lymphatic vessels called lacteals in the small intestine absorb dietary fats and fat-soluble vitamins (such as vitamins A, D, E, and K) from the digestive tract.
   - **Chyle Formation:** Fats absorbed by lacteals combine with lymphatic fluid to form a milky substance called chyle, which is transported through the lymphatic system to the bloodstream.
4. **Transportation of Immune Cells:**
   - **Migration of Immune Cells:** The lymphatic system facilitates the movement of immune cells, such as lymphocytes and dendritic cells, throughout the body. These cells travel via lymphatic vessels and lymph nodes, patrolling tissues and organs to detect and eliminate pathogens.

5. Removal of Cellular Waste and Toxins:
- **Clearance of Waste Products:** Lymphatic vessels collect cellular waste, toxins, and debris from tissues, helping to maintain tissue health and function.
- **Detoxification:** By removing metabolic waste and toxins, the lymphatic system supports the body's detoxification processes and promotes overall health.

6. Cancer Surveillance:
- **Metastasis Prevention:** Lymph nodes act as checkpoints for cancer cells, helping to prevent the spread of cancer (metastasis) by trapping and destroying cancerous cells before they can travel to other parts of the body.
- **Diagnostic Tool:** The examination of lymph nodes for cancer cells is an important diagnostic tool in cancer staging and treatment planning.

7. Regulation of Inflammatory Responses:
- **Resolution of Inflammation:** The lymphatic system helps to regulate inflammatory responses by removing inflammatory mediators and excess fluid from inflamed tissues, contributing to the resolution of inflammation and tissue repair.

Chapter 2: Principles of the Lymphatic Diet

Key Components of a Lymphatic Diet

A lymphatic diet focuses on supporting the health and function of the lymphatic system through specific dietary choices.

1. Hydration:
- Adequate hydration is crucial for maintaining lymphatic fluid volume and flow.
- Drink plenty of water throughout the day to support lymphatic drainage and detoxification.
- Herbal teas, such as green tea and dandelion tea, may also be beneficial for promoting lymphatic health.

2. Anti-inflammatory Foods:
- Emphasize a diet rich in fruits, vegetables, whole grains, and healthy fats.
- Choose foods high in antioxidants, such as berries, leafy greens, and citrus fruits, to reduce inflammation and support immune function.
- Include sources of healthy fats, such as avocados, olive oil, nuts, and seeds, to help combat inflammation and support lymphatic health.

3. Nutrient-Dense Foods:
- Consume foods rich in essential nutrients that support immune function and lymphatic health.
- Include sources of vitamin C (citrus fruits, bell peppers, strawberries), vitamin E (nuts, seeds, spinach), and omega-3 fatty acids (fatty fish, flaxseeds, walnuts).
- Ensure adequate intake of protein from sources such as lean meats, poultry, fish, legumes, and tofu to support immune cell production.

4. Lymphatic-Friendly Foods:
- Incorporate foods that promote lymphatic drainage and detoxification.
- Citrus fruits, leafy greens, cruciferous vegetables, and herbs like turmeric and ginger are particularly beneficial.

5. Herbal Supplements and Remedies:
- Consider incorporating herbal supplements and remedies that support lymphatic health.
- Turmeric, ginger, echinacea, and dandelion root are believed to have lymphatic-stimulating and immune-supportive properties.
- Consult with a healthcare professional before taking any herbal supplements, especially if you have underlying health conditions or are taking medications.

6. Avoidance of Inflammatory Substances:
- Limit or avoid processed foods, refined sugars, trans fats, and excessive alcohol, as these can promote inflammation and impair lymphatic function.
- Reduce intake of high-sodium foods, as excessive sodium can lead to fluid retention and lymphatic congestion.

7. Regular Physical Activity:
- Incorporate regular exercise into your routine to promote lymphatic circulation and drainage.
- Activities such as walking, jogging, swimming, yoga, and rebounding (mini trampoline exercises) can support lymphatic flow and overall lymphatic health.

8. Stress Management:
- Practice stress-reducing techniques such as meditation, deep breathing, yoga, and tai chi to support lymphatic health.
- Chronic stress can impair immune function and lymphatic circulation, so managing stress is essential for overall well-being.

In summary, a lymphatic diet focuses on nourishing the body with nutrient-dense, anti-inflammatory foods that support immune function and lymphatic health. By emphasizing hydration, consuming a variety of fruits and vegetables, incorporating lymphatic-friendly foods and herbs, and avoiding inflammatory substances, individuals can optimize their lymphatic system function and promote overall well-being. It's essential to consult with a healthcare professional or registered dietitian before making significant dietary changes, especially if you have underlying health conditions or dietary restrictions.

Foods to Embrace

1. **Fruits:**
   - **Citrus Fruits:** Oranges, lemons, limes, and grapefruits are rich in vitamin C and antioxidants, which support immune function and lymphatic health.
   - **Berries:** Blueberries, strawberries, raspberries, and blackberries are packed with antioxidants that help reduce inflammation and support detoxification.
   - **Pineapple:** Contains bromelain, an enzyme with anti-inflammatory properties that may aid in lymphatic drainage.
   - **Watermelon:** High water content and contains lycopene, an antioxidant that supports immune function.
   - **Kiwi:** Rich in vitamin C and fiber, which promote immune function and digestive health.
2. **Vegetables:**
   - **Leafy Greens:** Spinach, kale, Swiss chard, and collard greens are rich in chlorophyll, antioxidants, and fiber, which support detoxification and lymphatic health.
   - **Cruciferous Vegetables:** Broccoli, cauliflower, Brussels sprouts, and cabbage contain sulfur compounds that aid in detoxification and support immune function.
   - **Bell Peppers:** Rich in vitamin C and antioxidants, bell peppers support immune function and collagen production.
   - **Carrots:** High in beta-carotene, which converts to vitamin A in the body and supports immune function.
   - **Beets:** Contain betalains, antioxidants that support liver function and detoxification.
3. **Herbs and Spices:**
   - **Turmeric:** Contains curcumin, a potent anti-inflammatory compound that supports immune function and lymphatic health.
   - **Ginger:** Has anti-inflammatory properties and may aid in digestion and lymphatic circulation.

- **Garlic:** Contains allicin, a compound with immune-boosting and antimicrobial properties.
- **Cilantro:** Supports detoxification and may help remove heavy metals from the body.

4. Healthy Fats:
- **Avocado:** Rich in monounsaturated fats and antioxidants that support immune function and inflammation regulation.
- **Olive Oil:** Contains oleocanthal, an anti-inflammatory compound, and monounsaturated fats that support heart health.
- **Nuts and Seeds:** Almonds, walnuts, chia seeds, and flaxseeds are rich in omega-3 fatty acids and antioxidants that support immune function and inflammation regulation.

5. Lean Protein:
- **Poultry:** Chicken and turkey are excellent sources of lean protein that support immune function and tissue repair.
- **Fish:** Fatty fish like salmon, mackerel, and trout are rich in omega-3 fatty acids and protein, which support immune function and inflammation regulation.
- **Legumes:** Beans, lentils, and chickpeas are rich in protein, fiber, and antioxidants that support immune function and digestive health.

6. Probiotic Foods:
- **Yogurt:** Contains beneficial probiotics that support gut health and immune function.
- **Kefir:** A fermented dairy product rich in probiotics that support digestive health and immune function.
- **Sauerkraut:** Fermented cabbage that contains probiotics and supports gut health and immune function.

7. Hydrating Foods:
- **Cucumber:** High water content and contains silica, which supports connective tissue health.
- **Celery:** High water content and contains electrolytes that support hydration and fluid balance.

Foods to Avoid.

1. **Processed Foods:**
   - **Fast Food:** High in unhealthy fats, sodium, and additives that can contribute to inflammation and lymphatic congestion.
   - **Packaged Snacks:** Chips, cookies, and other processed snacks are often high in refined sugars, trans fats, and artificial ingredients that can disrupt lymphatic function.
2. **Refined Sugars and Sweets:**
   - **Soda:** High in sugar and artificial additives, soda can contribute to inflammation and lymphatic congestion.
   - **Candy:** High in refined sugars and artificial ingredients that can negatively impact immune function and overall health.
   - **Desserts:** Cakes, pastries, and other desserts often contain high levels of refined sugars, unhealthy fats, and additives that can contribute to inflammation and lymphatic congestion.
3. **Trans Fats and Hydrogenated Oils:**
   - **Fried Foods:** French fries, fried chicken, and other fried foods are high in trans fats and unhealthy oils that can promote inflammation and lymphatic congestion.
   - **Commercial Baked Goods:** Doughnuts, muffins, and other baked goods often contain hydrogenated oils, which can negatively impact heart health and immune function.
4. **High-Sodium Foods:**
   - **Processed Meats:** Bacon, sausage, and deli meats are high in sodium and preservatives that can contribute to fluid retention and lymphatic congestion.
   - **Canned Soups:** Often high in sodium, canned soups can contribute to fluid retention and lymphatic congestion.
   - **Salty Snacks:** Potato chips, pretzels, and salted nuts are high in sodium and can contribute to fluid retention and lymphatic congestion.
5. **Alcohol:**
   - ****Excessive alcohol consumption can dehydrate the body and impair lymphatic function.
   - **Alcoholic Beverages:** Beer, wine, and liquor can contribute to inflammation and lymphatic congestion when consumed in excess.

6. **Dairy Products:**
   - **High-Fat Dairy:** Whole milk, cheese, and ice cream are high in saturated fats and can contribute to inflammation and lymphatic congestion.
   - **Processed Dairy:** Flavored yogurt, sweetened milk alternatives, and other processed dairy products may contain added sugars and additives that can negatively impact lymphatic health.
7. **Gluten and Wheat:**
   - **Processed Wheat Products:** White bread, pasta, and baked goods made from refined wheat flour can contribute to inflammation and lymphatic congestion.
   - **Gluten-Containing Foods:** Some individuals may be sensitive to gluten, a protein found in wheat, barley, and rye, which can contribute to inflammation and lymphatic congestion in susceptible individuals.

Avoiding processed foods, refined sugars, trans fats, high-sodium foods, alcohol, dairy products, and gluten-containing foods can support lymphatic health, reduce inflammation, and promote overall well-being. Instead, focus on whole, nutrient-dense foods that support immune function, detoxification, and lymphatic drainage. It's essential to listen to your body and make dietary choices that support your individual health needs and goals. Consulting with a healthcare professional or registered dietitian can provide personalized guidance and support for optimizing your lymphatic diet.

BREKFAST RECIPES

1. Coconut Chia Pudding

Ingredients:
- 1/4 cup chia seeds
- 1 cup coconut milk
- 1 tablespoon maple syrup (optional)
- 1/2 teaspoon vanilla extract
- Fresh berries for topping (optional)

Instructions:
1. In a mixing bowl, combine chia seeds, coconut milk, maple syrup (if using), and vanilla extract.
2. Stir well to combine all ingredients thoroughly.
3. Cover the bowl and refrigerate for at least 2 hours or overnight, allowing the chia seeds to absorb the liquid and thicken.
4. Stir the pudding mixture once more before serving.
5. Serve chilled, topped with fresh berries if desired.

Nutritional Information:
- Serving Size: 1/2 cup
- Servings: 2
- Calories per serving: approximately 180
- Total Fat: 12g
- Carbohydrates: 14g
- Fiber: 9g
- Protein: 5g

Cooking Time:
- Prep Time: 5 minutes
- Refrigeration Time: 2 hours or overnight

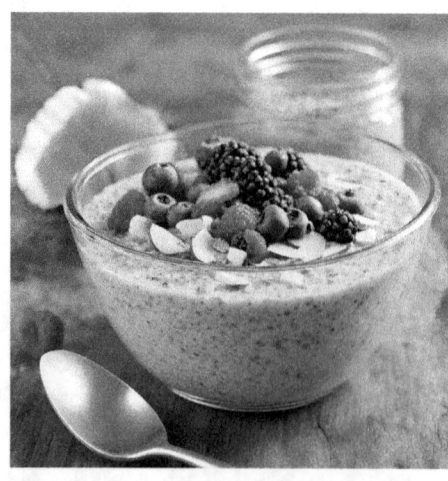

2. Tofu Scramble

Ingredients:
- 1 block firm tofu, drained and crumbled
- 1 tablespoon olive oil
- 1/2 onion, diced
- 1 bell pepper, diced
- 1/2 teaspoon turmeric
- Salt and pepper to taste
- Fresh parsley for garnish (optional)

Instructions:
1. Heat olive oil in a skillet over medium heat.
2. Add diced onion and bell pepper to the skillet and sauté until softened.
3. Add crumbled tofu to the skillet, along with turmeric, salt, and pepper.
4. Cook, stirring occasionally, for about 5-7 minutes, or until the tofu is heated through and slightly browned.
5. Garnish with fresh parsley if desired before serving.

Nutritional Information:
- Serving Size: 1/2 cup
- Servings: 4
- Calories per serving: approximately 120
- Total Fat: 7g
- Carbohydrates: 5g
- Fiber: 2g
- Protein: 10g

Cooking Time:
- Prep Time: 10 minutes
- Cooking Time: 10 minutes

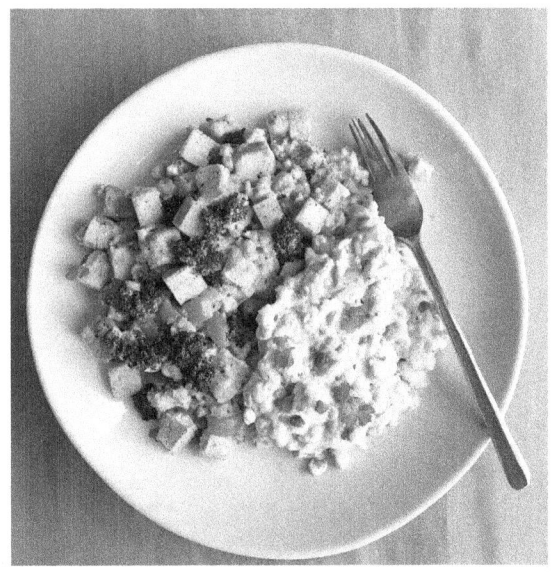

3. Greek Yogurt with Nuts and Seeds

Ingredients:
- 1 cup Greek yogurt
- 1 tablespoon honey or maple syrup (optional)
- 2 tablespoons mixed nuts (such as almonds, walnuts, or pecans), chopped
- 1 tablespoon mixed seeds (such as chia seeds, flaxseeds, or pumpkin seeds)

Instructions:
1. In a serving bowl, spoon Greek yogurt.
2. Drizzle honey or maple syrup over the yogurt if desired.
3. Sprinkle chopped nuts and seeds over the yogurt.
4. Serve immediately.

Nutritional Information:
- Serving Size: 1/2 cup
- Servings: 2
- Calories per serving: approximately 150 (without honey/maple syrup)
- Total Fat: 10g
- Carbohydrates: 7g
- Fiber: 2g
- Protein: 10g

Cooking Time:
- Prep Time: 5 minutes

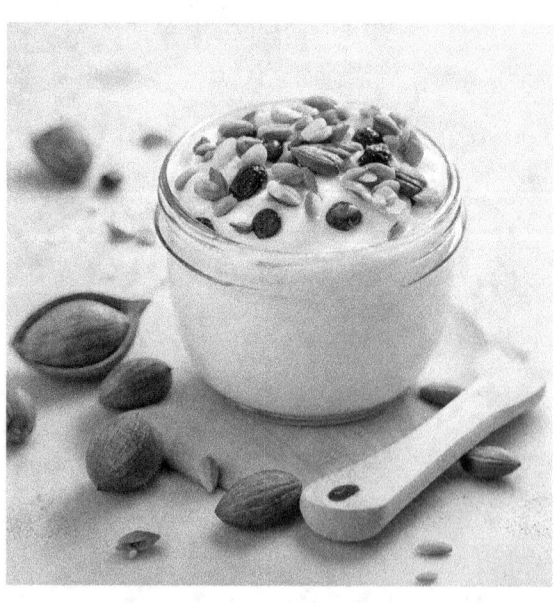

4. Almond Butter Banana Wrap

Ingredients:
- 1 whole wheat tortilla
- 2 tablespoons almond butter
- 1 banana, thinly sliced
- 1 teaspoon honey (optional)
- Cinnamon for sprinkling (optional)

Instructions:
1. Spread almond butter evenly over the whole wheat tortilla.
2. Place thinly sliced banana on top of the almond butter.
3. Drizzle honey over the banana slices if desired.
4. Sprinkle cinnamon over the banana slices if desired.
5. Roll up the tortilla tightly.
6. Slice the wrap in half or into bite-sized pieces if preferred.
7. Serve immediately or wrap in parchment paper for later.

Nutritional Information:
- Serving Size: 1 wrap
- Servings: 1
- Calories per serving: approximately 350
- Total Fat: 15g
- Carbohydrates: 50g
- Fiber: 8g
- Protein: 9g

Cooking Time:
- Prep Time: 5 minutes

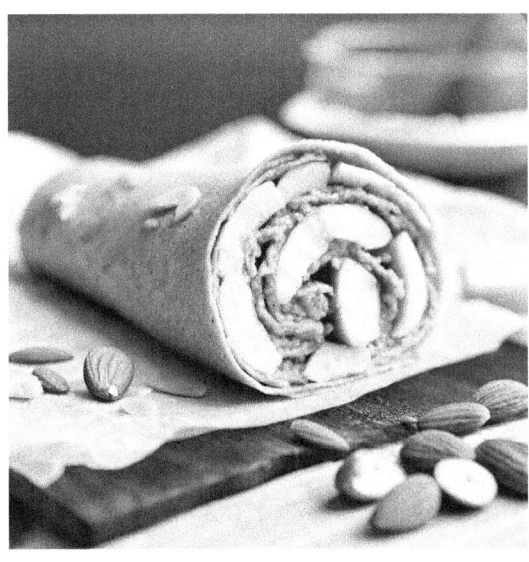

5. Beetroot Smoothie

Ingredients:
- 1 small beetroot, peeled and diced
- 1 cup frozen mixed berries
- 1 ripe banana
- 1 cup spinach leaves
- 1 cup almond milk (or any preferred milk)
- 1 tablespoon honey (optional)
- Ice cubes (optional)

Instructions:
1. Place all ingredients in a blender.
2. Blend until smooth and creamy.
3. Add ice cubes if desired for a colder smoothie.
4. Pour into glasses and serve immediately.

Nutritional Information:
- Serving Size: 1 cup
- Servings: 2
- Calories per serving: approximately 150
- Total Fat: 2g
- Carbohydrates: 32g
- Fiber: 7g
- Protein: 3g

Cooking Time:
- Prep Time: 5 minutes

6. Cinnamon Apple Oatmeal

Ingredients:
- 1 cup rolled oats
- 2 cups water or milk of choice
- 1 apple, diced
- 1 tablespoon honey or maple syrup
- 1/2 teaspoon ground cinnamon
- 1/4 cup chopped nuts (optional)
- Fresh apple slices for garnish (optional)

Instructions:
1. In a saucepan, bring water or milk to a boil.
2. Stir in rolled oats, diced apple, honey or maple syrup, and ground cinnamon.
3. Reduce heat to low and simmer for about 5-7 minutes, stirring occasionally, until oats are cooked and creamy.
4. Remove from heat and stir in chopped nuts if using.
5. Serve hot, garnished with fresh apple slices if desired.

Nutritional Information:
- Serving Size: 1 cup
- Servings: 2
- Calories per serving: approximately 250
- Total Fat: 5g
- Carbohydrates: 45g
- Fiber: 7g
- Protein: 7g

Cooking Time:
- Prep Time: 5 minutes
- Cooking Time: 10 minutes

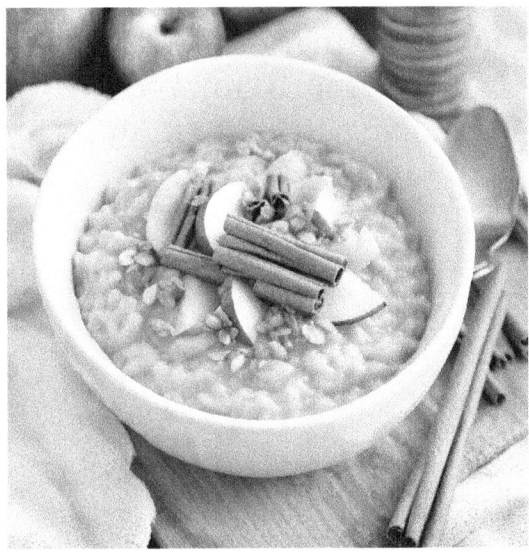

7. Breakfast Tacos

Ingredients:
- 4 small whole wheat tortillas
- 4 eggs
- 1/2 cup black beans, drained and rinsed
- 1/2 avocado, sliced
- 1/4 cup salsa
- Salt and pepper to taste
- Fresh cilantro for garnish (optional)

Instructions:
1. Heat a skillet over medium heat and scramble the eggs.
2. Warm the tortillas in the skillet or microwave.
3. Divide scrambled eggs among the tortillas.
4. Top each with black beans, avocado slices, salsa, salt, and pepper.
5. Garnish with fresh cilantro if desired.
6. Serve immediately.

Nutritional Information:
- Serving Size: 1 taco
- Servings: 4
- Calories per serving: approximately 250
- Total Fat: 10g
- Carbohydrates: 25g
- Fiber: 6g
- Protein: 15g

Cooking Time:
- Prep Time: 10 minutes
- Cooking Time: 10 minutes

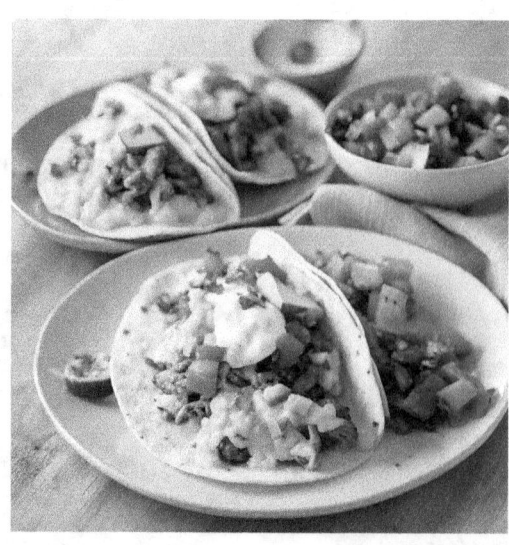

8. Zucchini Fritters

Ingredients:
- 2 medium zucchinis, grated
- 1/2 teaspoon salt
- 1/4 cup whole wheat flour
- 1 egg
- 1/4 cup grated Parmesan cheese
- 2 tablespoons chopped fresh parsley
- 1 clove garlic, minced
- 2 tablespoons olive oil

Instructions:
1. Place grated zucchini in a colander and sprinkle with salt. Let sit for 10 minutes, then squeeze out excess moisture.
2. In a mixing bowl, combine grated zucchini, whole wheat flour, egg, Parmesan cheese, parsley, and minced garlic. Mix until well combined.
3. Heat olive oil in a skillet over medium heat.
4. Scoop spoonfuls of the zucchini mixture into the skillet, flattening them slightly with the back of the spoon.
5. Cook for 3-4 minutes on each side, or until golden brown and cooked through.
6. Remove from skillet and place on a plate lined with paper towels to drain excess oil.
7. Serve warm.

Nutritional Information:
- Serving Size: 2 fritters
- Servings: 4
- Calories per serving: approximately 150
- Total Fat: 9g
- Carbohydrates: 10g
- Fiber: 2g
- Protein: 6g

Cooking Time:
- Prep Time: 15 minutes
- Cooking Time: 10 minutes

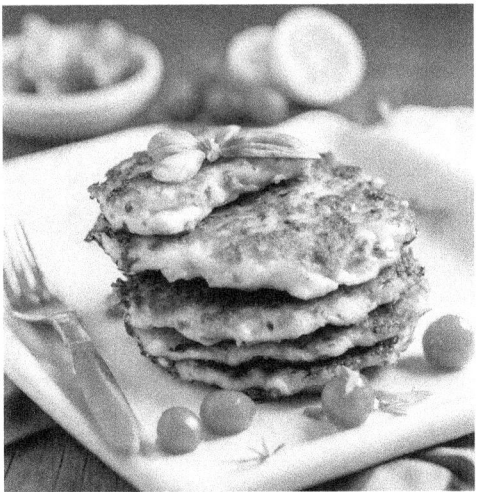

9. Acai Bowl

Ingredients:
- 2 packets frozen acai puree
- 1 ripe banana
- 1/2 cup frozen mixed berries
- 1/2 cup almond milk (or any preferred milk)
- Toppings: sliced banana, granola, shredded coconut, chia seeds, sliced almonds, honey or maple syrup

Instructions:
1. In a blender, combine acai puree, banana, frozen mixed berries, and almond milk.
2. Blend until smooth and creamy.
3. Pour the smoothie into bowls.
4. Top with sliced banana, granola, shredded coconut, chia seeds, sliced almonds, and a drizzle of honey or maple syrup.
5. Serve immediately.

Nutritional Information:
- Serving Size: 1 bowl
- Servings: 2
- Calories per serving: approximately 250
- Total Fat: 8g
- Carbohydrates: 40g
- Fiber: 9g
- Protein: 5g

Cooking Time:
- Prep Time: 5 minutes

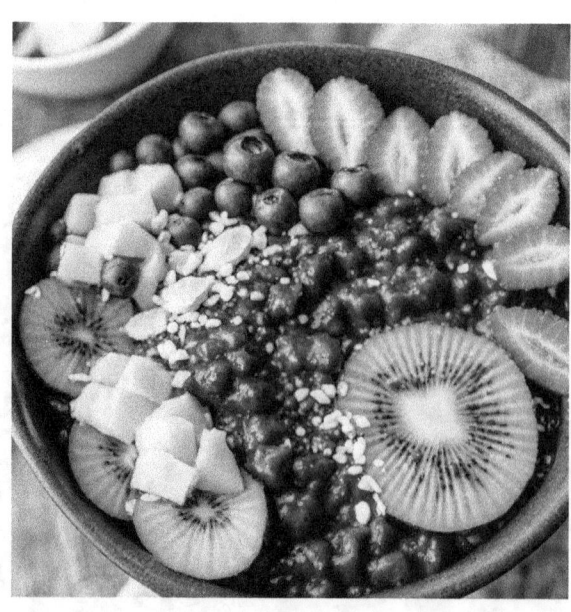

10. Spinach and Feta Crustless Quiche

Ingredients:
- 6 eggs
- 1 cup spinach, chopped
- 1/2 cup crumbled feta cheese
- 1/4 cup diced tomatoes
- 1/4 cup diced bell peppers
- Salt and pepper to taste

Instructions:
1. Preheat the oven to 350°F (175°C) and grease a pie dish.
2. In a mixing bowl, whisk together eggs, chopped spinach, crumbled feta cheese, diced tomatoes, diced bell peppers, salt, and pepper.
3. Pour the mixture into the prepared pie dish.
4. Bake in the preheated oven for 25-30 minutes, or until the quiche is set and golden brown on top.
5. Remove from the oven and let it cool for a few minutes before slicing.
6. Serve warm or at room temperature.

Nutritional Information:
- Serving Size: 1 slice
- Servings: 6
- Calories per serving: approximately 120
- Total Fat: 8g
- Carbohydrates: 2g
- Fiber: 1g
- Protein: 10g

Cooking Time:
- Prep Time: 10 minutes
- Baking Time: 25-30 minutes

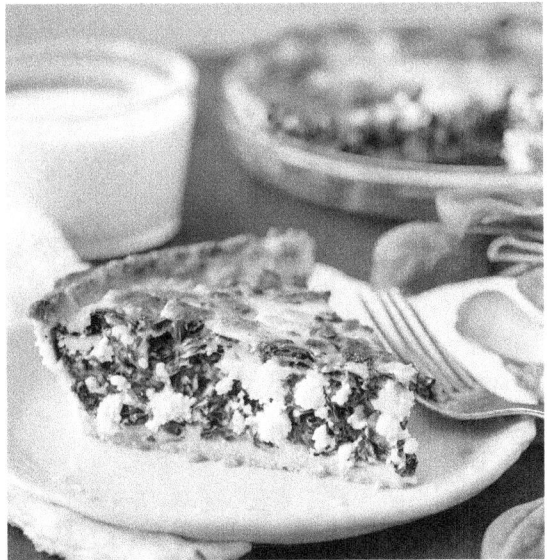

11. Fruit Salad

Ingredients (continued):
- 1 tablespoon honey or maple syrup
- Juice of 1/2 lemon
- Fresh mint leaves for garnish (optional)

Instructions:
1. In a large mixing bowl, combine the diced mixed fruits.
2. Drizzle honey or maple syrup over the fruits.
3. Squeeze the lemon juice over the fruits.
4. Gently toss the fruits until they are evenly coated with the honey/maple syrup and lemon juice.
5. Transfer the fruit salad to a serving dish.
6. Garnish with fresh mint leaves if desired.
7. Serve chilled.

Nutritional Information:
- Serving Size: 1 cup
- Servings: 4
- Calories per serving: approximately 80
- Total Fat: 0g
- Carbohydrates: 20g
- Fiber: 3g
- Protein: 1g

Cooking Time:
- Prep Time: 10 minutes

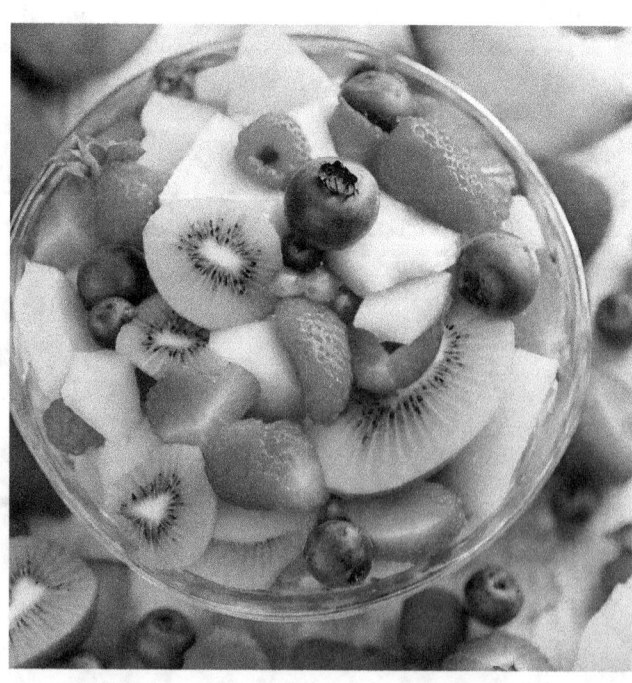

12. Cauliflower Hash Browns

Ingredients:
- 1 small head cauliflower, grated
- 1/4 cup grated Parmesan cheese
- 1 egg, beaten
- 1/4 teaspoon garlic powder
- 1/4 teaspoon onion powder
- Salt and pepper to taste
- 2 tablespoons olive oil

Instructions:
1. Preheat the oven to 400°F (200°C). Line a baking sheet with parchment paper.
2. In a large mixing bowl, combine grated cauliflower, grated Parmesan cheese, beaten egg, garlic powder, onion powder, salt, and pepper. Mix until well combined.
3. Using your hands, shape the cauliflower mixture into small patties.
4. Place the patties on the prepared baking sheet.
5. Brush the tops of the patties with olive oil.
6. Bake in the preheated oven for 20-25 minutes, flipping halfway through, or until the hash browns are golden brown and crispy.
7. Remove from the oven and let them cool slightly before serving.
8. Serve warm.

Nutritional Information:
- Serving Size: 2 hash browns
- Servings: 4
- Calories per serving: approximately 100
- Total Fat: 7g
- Carbohydrates: 6g
- Fiber: 3g
- Protein: 4g

Cooking Time:
- Prep Time: 15 minutes
- Baking Time: 20-25 minutes

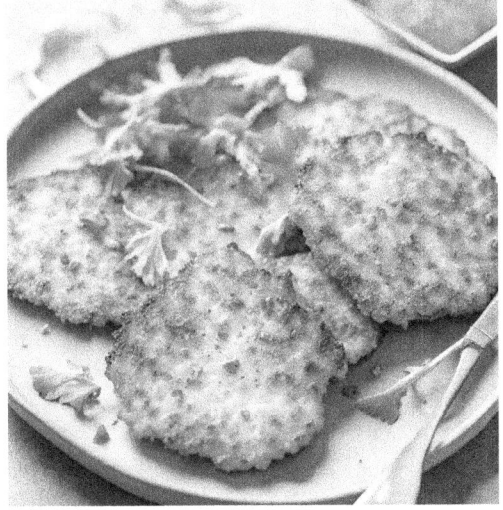

13. Lentil Porridge

Ingredients:
- 1 cup red lentils
- 2 cups water or vegetable broth
- 1/2 teaspoon ground turmeric
- 1/2 teaspoon ground cumin
- Salt and pepper to taste
- Optional toppings: sliced avocado, chopped fresh herbs, toasted nuts or seeds

Instructions:
1. Rinse the lentils under cold water until the water runs clear.
2. In a medium saucepan, combine the rinsed lentils, water or vegetable broth, ground turmeric, and ground cumin.
3. Bring the mixture to a boil, then reduce the heat to low and simmer for about 15-20 minutes, or until the lentils are soft and the mixture has thickened to a porridge-like consistency.
4. Season with salt and pepper to taste.
5. Serve hot, topped with your choice of optional toppings.

Nutritional Information:
- Serving Size: 1 cup
- Servings: 2
- Calories per serving: approximately 200
- Total Fat: 1g
- Carbohydrates: 36g
- Fiber: 15g
- Protein: 14g

Cooking Time:
- Prep Time: 5 minutes
- Cooking Time: 20-25 minutes

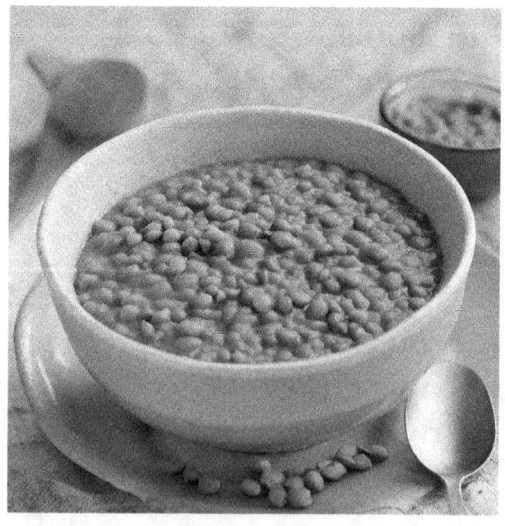

14. Veggie Breakfast Burrito

Ingredients:
- 4 whole wheat tortillas
- 4 eggs, scrambled
- 1/2 cup black beans, drained and rinsed
- 1/2 cup diced bell peppers
- 1/4 cup diced onions
- 1/4 cup shredded cheddar cheese (optional)
- Salt and pepper to taste
- Salsa or hot sauce for serving (optional)

Instructions:
1. Heat a skillet over medium heat and scramble the eggs.
2. Warm the whole wheat tortillas in the skillet or microwave.
3. Divide the scrambled eggs, black beans, diced bell peppers, diced onions, and shredded cheddar cheese (if using) among the tortillas.
4. Season with salt and pepper to taste.
5. Roll up the tortillas, folding in the sides to secure the filling.
6. Serve hot, with salsa or hot sauce if desired.

Nutritional Information:
- Serving Size: 1 burrito
- Servings: 4
- Calories per serving: approximately 250
- Total Fat: 8g
- Carbohydrates: 30g
- Fiber: 6g
- Protein: 15g

Cooking Time:
- Prep Time: 10 minutes
- Cooking Time: 10 minutes

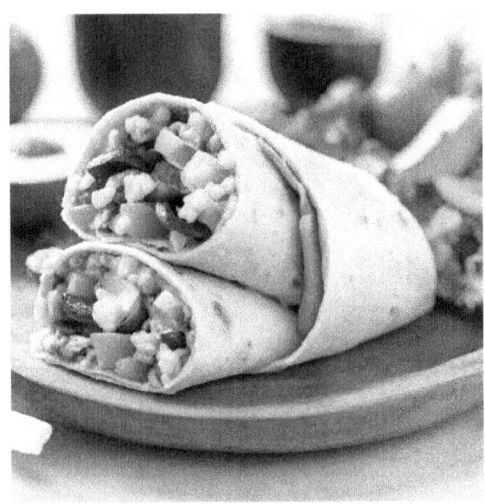

15. Sweet Potato Toast

Ingredients:
- 1 large sweet potato, sliced lengthwise into 1/4-inch thick slices
- Toppings of your choice: avocado slices, mashed avocado, almond butter, sliced banana, berries, etc.

Instructions:
1. Preheat the oven to 400°F (200°C). Line a baking sheet with parchment paper.
2. Place the sweet potato slices on the prepared baking sheet.
3. Bake in the preheated oven for 20-25 minutes, flipping halfway through, or until the sweet potato slices are tender and lightly browned.
4. Remove from the oven and let them cool slightly.
5. Top with your choice of toppings.
6. Serve immediately.

Nutritional Information:
- Serving Size: 1 sweet potato slice (without toppings)
- Servings: Depends on the size of the sweet potato
- Calories per serving: approximately 50
- Total Fat: 0g
- Carbohydrates: 12g
- Fiber: 2g
- Protein: 1g

Cooking Time:
- Prep Time: 5 minutes
- Baking Time: 20-25 minutes

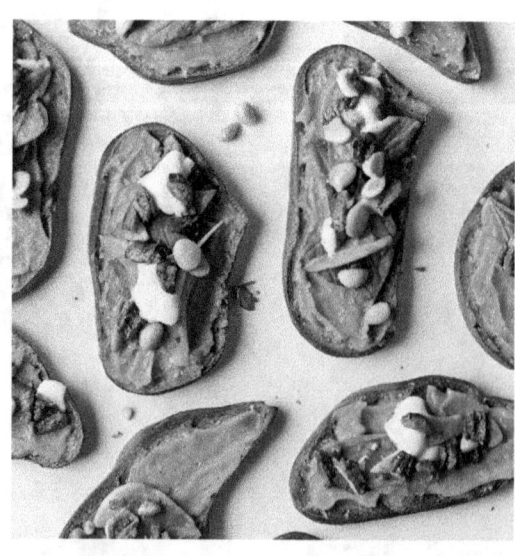

16. Buckwheat Pancakes

Ingredients:
- 1 cup buckwheat flour
- 1 tablespoon ground flaxseeds
- 1 teaspoon baking powder
- 1/4 teaspoon ground cinnamon
- 1 cup almond milk (or any preferred milk)
- 1 tablespoon maple syrup
- 1 teaspoon vanilla extract
- Cooking spray or oil for greasing the skillet

Instructions:
1. In a mixing bowl, whisk together buckwheat flour, ground flaxseeds, baking powder, and ground cinnamon.
2. In a separate bowl, combine almond milk, maple syrup, and vanilla extract.
3. Pour the wet ingredients into the dry ingredients and mix until well combined.
4. Heat a skillet or griddle over medium heat and lightly grease with cooking spray or oil.
5. Pour 1/4 cup of batter onto the skillet for each pancake.
6. Cook for 2-3 minutes on each side, or until golden brown and cooked through.
7. Repeat with the remaining batter.
8. Serve warm with your choice of toppings.

Nutritional Information:
- Serving Size: 2 pancakes
- Servings: 4
- Calories per serving: approximately 150
- Total Fat: 2g
- Carbohydrates: 28g
- Fiber: 4g
- Protein: 5g

Cooking Time:
- Prep Time: 10 minutes
- Cooking Time: 10 minutes

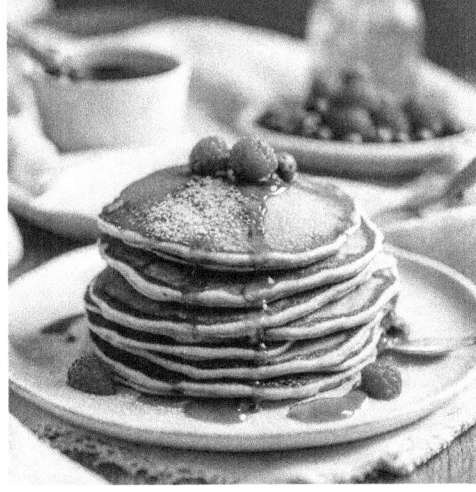

17. Coconut Yogurt Parfait

Ingredients:
- 1 cup coconut yogurt
- 1/2 cup granola
- 1/2 cup mixed berries (such as strawberries, blueberries, raspberries)
- 2 tablespoons shredded coconut

Instructions:
1. In a glass or bowl, layer coconut yogurt, granola, mixed berries, and shredded coconut.
2. Repeat the layers until all ingredients are used, ending with a layer of mixed berries and shredded coconut on top.
3. Serve immediately as a healthy breakfast or snack option.

Nutritional Information:
- Serving Size: 1 parfait
- Servings: 2
- Calories per serving: approximately 250
- Total Fat: 10g
- Carbohydrates: 35g
- Fiber: 5g
- Protein: 7g

Cooking Time:
- Prep Time: 5 minutes

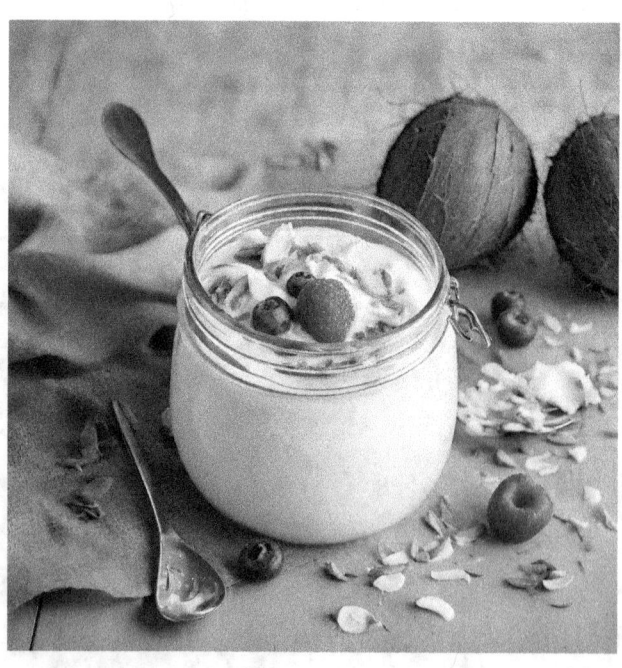

18. Vegetable Omelette

Ingredients:
- 4 eggs
- 1/4 cup diced bell peppers
- 1/4 cup diced onions
- 1/4 cup diced tomatoes
- 1/4 cup chopped spinach leaves
- Salt and pepper to taste
- 1 tablespoon olive oil

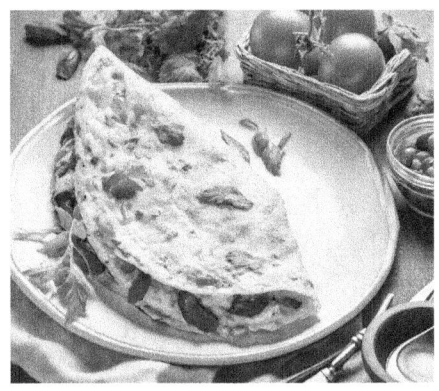

Instructions:
1. In a mixing bowl, beat the eggs until well combined.
2. Heat olive oil in a skillet over medium heat.
3. Add diced bell peppers, onions, and tomatoes to the skillet. Cook until softened.
4. Add chopped spinach leaves to the skillet and cook until wilted.
5. Pour the beaten eggs over the vegetables in the skillet.
6. Cook for 2-3 minutes, or until the edges start to set.
7. Use a spatula to gently lift the edges of the omelette and tilt the skillet to allow the uncooked eggs to flow to the bottom.
8. Continue cooking until the omelette is set but still slightly moist on top.
9. Season with salt and pepper to taste.
10. Carefully fold the omelette over, covering the vegetables.
11. Cook for another minute until the omelette is fully cooked through.
12. Slide the omelette onto a plate and fold it in half.
13. Serve hot with a side of fresh salad or whole wheat toast.

Nutritional Information:
- Serving Size: 1 omelette
- Servings: 2
- Calories per serving: approximately 200
- Total Fat: 14g
- Carbohydrates: 8g
- Fiber: 2g
- Protein: 12g

Cooking Time:
- Prep Time: 10 minutes
- Cooking Time: 10 minutes

19. Berry Smoothie

Ingredients:
- 1 cup mixed berries (such as strawberries, blueberries, raspberries)
- 1 ripe banana
- 1/2 cup plain Greek yogurt
- 1/2 cup almond milk (or any preferred milk)
- 1 tablespoon honey or maple syrup (optional)
- Ice cubes (optional)

Instructions:
1. Place all ingredients in a blender.
2. Blend until smooth and creamy.
3. Add ice cubes if desired for a colder smoothie.
4. Pour into glasses and serve immediately.

Nutritional Information:
- Serving Size: 1 cup
- Servings: 2
- Calories per serving: approximately 150
- Total Fat: 1g
- Carbohydrates: 30g
- Fiber: 5g
- Protein: 7g

Cooking Time:
- Prep Time: 5 minutes

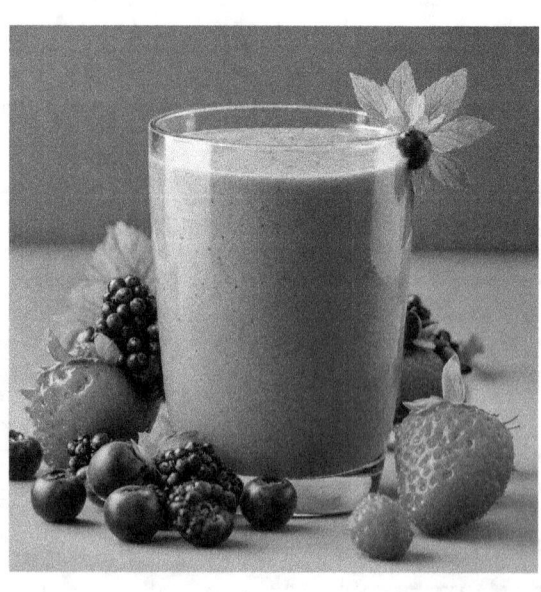

20. Turmeric Scrambled Eggs

Ingredients:
- 4 eggs
- 1/2 teaspoon ground turmeric
- Salt and pepper to taste
- 1 tablespoon olive oil
- Fresh parsley for garnish (optional)

Instructions:
1. In a mixing bowl, beat the eggs until well combined.
2. Add ground turmeric, salt, and pepper to the beaten eggs and mix well.
3. Heat olive oil in a skillet over medium heat.
4. Pour the egg mixture into the skillet.
5. Cook, stirring occasionally, until the eggs are scrambled and cooked to your desired consistency.
6. Remove from heat and transfer to a serving plate.
7. Garnish with fresh parsley if desired.
8. Serve hot.

Nutritional Information:
- Serving Size: 2 eggs
- Servings: 2
- Calories per serving: approximately 160
- Total Fat: 12g
- Carbohydrates: 1g
- Fiber: 0g
- Protein: 12g

Cooking Time:
- Prep Time: 5 minutes
- Cooking Time: 5 minutes

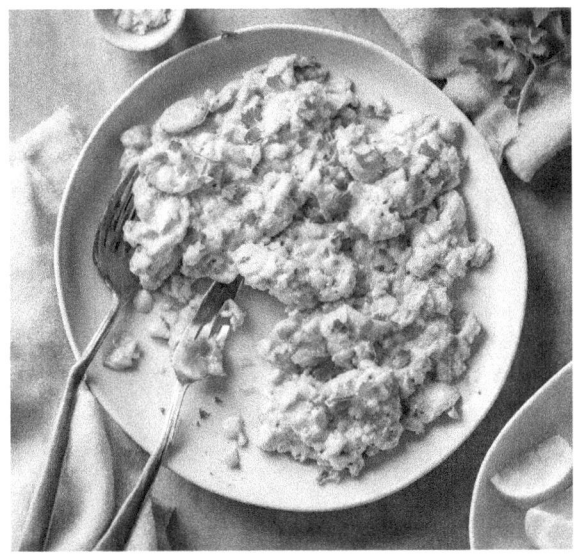

21. Green Smoothie Bowl

Ingredients:
- 1 ripe banana
- 1 cup spinach leaves
- 1/2 cup frozen mango chunks
- 1/2 cup frozen pineapple chunks
- 1/2 cup almond milk (or any preferred milk)
- Toppings: sliced kiwi, granola, shredded coconut, chia seeds, sliced almonds

Instructions:
1. In a blender, combine banana, spinach leaves, frozen mango chunks, frozen pineapple chunks, and almond milk.
2. Blend until smooth and creamy.
3. Pour the smoothie into a bowl.
4. Top with sliced kiwi, granola, shredded coconut, chia seeds, sliced almonds, or any other desired toppings.
5. Serve immediately with a spoon.

Nutritional Information:
- Serving Size: 1 bowl
- Servings: 1
- Calories per serving: approximately 350
- Total Fat: 10g
- Carbohydrates: 60g
- Fiber: 10g
- Protein: 8g

Cooking Time:
- Prep Time: 5 minutes

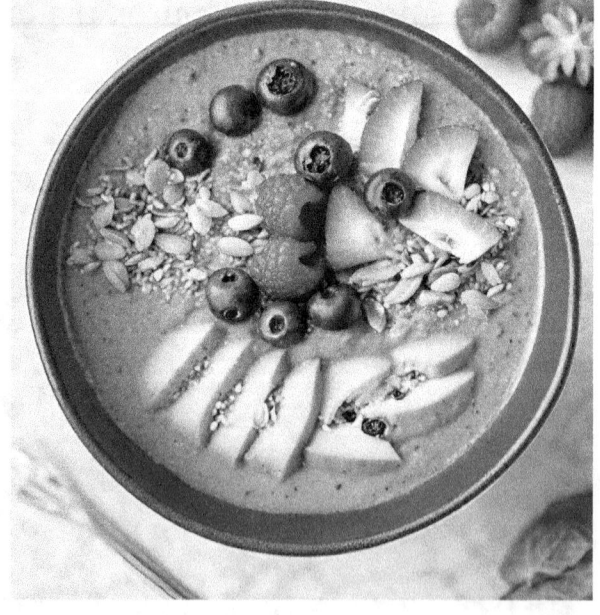

VEGETABLES

1. Grilled Asparagus with Lemon Zest
Ingredients:
- 1 bunch asparagus, trimmed
- 1 tablespoon olive oil
- Zest of 1 lemon
- Salt and pepper to taste

Instructions:
1. Preheat grill to medium-high heat.
2. In a bowl, toss asparagus with olive oil, lemon zest, salt, and pepper until evenly coated.
3. Place asparagus on the grill and cook for 3-4 minutes per side, or until tender and slightly charred.
4. Remove from grill and transfer to a serving platter.
5. Serve hot.

Nutritional Information:
- Serving Size: 1/2 cup
- Servings: 4
- Calories per serving: approximately 35
- Total Fat: 2g
- Carbohydrates: 4g
- Fiber: 2g
- Protein: 2g

Cooking Time:
- Prep Time: 5 minutes
- Cooking Time: 8-10 minutes

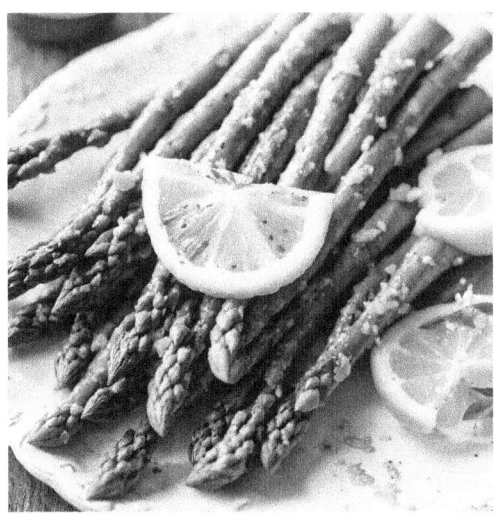

2. Korean Spinach Side Dish (Sigeumchi Namul)

Ingredients:
- 1 bunch spinach, washed and trimmed
- 2 cloves garlic, minced
- 1 tablespoon soy sauce
- 1 teaspoon sesame oil
- 1 teaspoon sesame seeds
- Salt to taste

Instructions:
1. Blanch the spinach in boiling water for 1 minute. Drain and rinse under cold water to stop the cooking process. Squeeze out excess water and chop.
2. In a skillet, heat sesame oil over medium heat. Add minced garlic and sauté until fragrant.
3. Add chopped spinach to the skillet and stir-fry for 2-3 minutes.
4. Stir in soy sauce and continue to cook for another minute.
5. Remove from heat and transfer to a serving dish.
6. Sprinkle sesame seeds on top.
7. Serve warm or at room temperature.

Nutritional Information:
- Serving Size: 1/2 cup
- Servings: 4
- Calories per serving: approximately 25
- Total Fat: 1.5g
- Carbohydrates: 2g
- Fiber: 1g
- Protein: 2g

Cooking Time:
- Prep Time: 10 minutes
- Cooking Time: 5 minutes

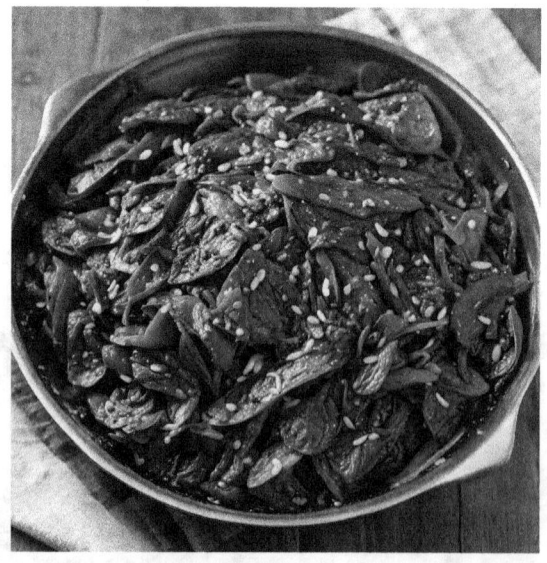

3. Swiss Chard Rolls

Ingredients:
- 8 large Swiss chard leaves
- 1 cup cooked quinoa
- 1/2 cup diced tomatoes
- 1/4 cup chopped olives
- 1/4 cup crumbled feta cheese
- 2 tablespoons chopped fresh parsley
- Salt and pepper to taste
- Lemon wedges for serving

Instructions:
1. Preheat oven to 375°F (190°C). Grease a baking dish.
2. Blanch Swiss chard leaves in boiling water for 1 minute. Remove and pat dry with paper towels.
3. In a bowl, mix cooked quinoa, diced tomatoes, chopped olives, crumbled feta cheese, chopped fresh parsley, salt, and pepper.
4. Place a spoonful of the quinoa mixture onto each Swiss chard leaf. Roll up and place seam-side down in the prepared baking dish.
5. Bake in the preheated oven for 15-20 minutes, or until heated through.
6. Serve hot with lemon wedges on the side.

Nutritional Information:
- Serving Size: 2 rolls
- Servings: 4
- Calories per serving: approximately 150
- Total Fat: 5g
- Carbohydrates: 20g
- Fiber: 5g
- Protein: 7g

Cooking Time:
- Prep Time: 20 minutes
- Cooking Time: 20 minutes

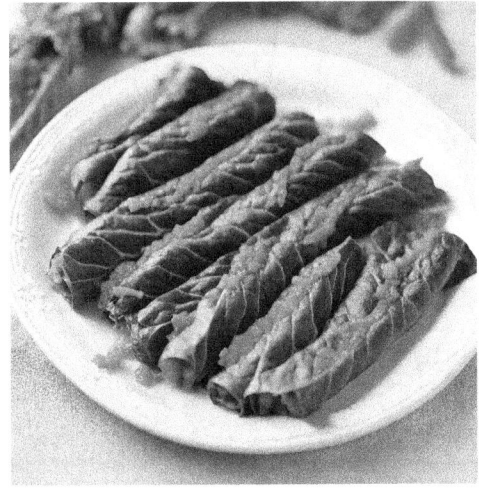

4. Szechuan Green Beans

Ingredients:
- 1 pound green beans, trimmed
- 2 tablespoons soy sauce
- 1 tablespoon rice vinegar
- 1 tablespoon hoisin sauce
- 1 tablespoon sesame oil
- 2 cloves garlic, minced
- 1 teaspoon grated ginger
- 1 tablespoon vegetable oil
- 1 teaspoon red pepper flakes (adjust to taste)
- Sesame seeds for garnish (optional)

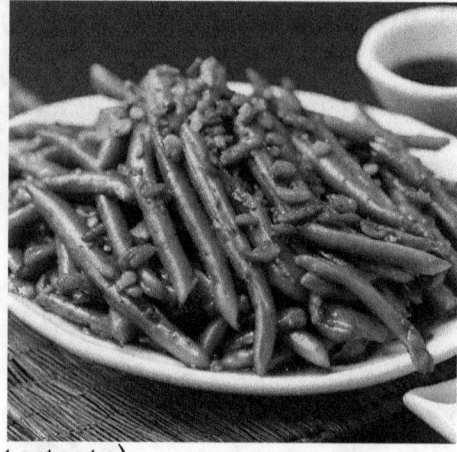

Instructions:
1. In a small bowl, whisk together soy sauce, rice vinegar, hoisin sauce, and sesame oil to make the sauce.
2. Heat vegetable oil in a skillet over medium-high heat. Add minced garlic and grated ginger, and cook for 1 minute until fragrant.
3. Add green beans to the skillet and stir-fry for 4-5 minutes until tender-crisp.
4. Pour the sauce over the green beans and toss to coat evenly.
5. Add red pepper flakes and continue to cook for another 1-2 minutes.
6. Remove from heat and transfer to a serving dish.
7. Garnish with sesame seeds if desired.
8. Serve hot.

Nutritional Information:
- Serving Size: 1/2 cup
- Servings: 6
- Calories per serving: approximately 60
- Total Fat: 4g
- Carbohydrates: 6g
- Fiber: 2g
- Protein: 2g

Cooking Time:
- Prep Time: 10 minutes
- Cooking Time: 10 minutes

5. Cabbage Stir-Fry

Ingredients:

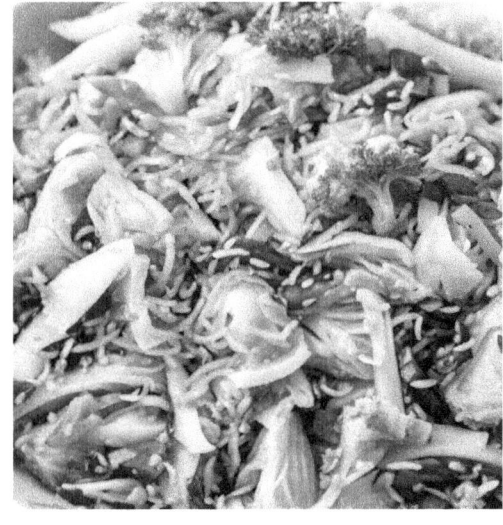

- 4 cups shredded cabbage
- 1 carrot, julienned
- 1 bell pepper, thinly sliced
- 2 cloves garlic, minced
- 1 tablespoon soy sauce
- 1 tablespoon rice vinegar
- 1 teaspoon sesame oil
- 1 teaspoon grated ginger
- 1 tablespoon vegetable oil
- Salt and pepper to taste
- Green onions for garnish (optional)

Instructions:

1. Heat vegetable oil in a large skillet or wok over medium-high heat.
2. Add minced garlic and grated ginger, and cook for 1 minute until fragrant.
3. Add shredded cabbage, julienned carrot, and sliced bell pepper to the skillet. Stir-fry for 4-5 minutes until vegetables are tender-crisp.
4. In a small bowl, whisk together soy sauce, rice vinegar, and sesame oil. Pour the sauce over the vegetables and toss to coat evenly.
5. Season with salt and pepper to taste.
6. Remove from heat and transfer to a serving dish.
7. Garnish with chopped green onions if desired.
8. Serve hot.

Nutritional Information:

- Serving Size: 1 cup
- Servings: 4
- Calories per serving: approximately 70
- Total Fat: 4g
- Carbohydrates: 8g
- Fiber: 3g
- Protein: 2g

Cooking Time:

- Prep Time: 10 minutes
- Cooking Time: 10 minutes

6. Spinach and Feta Stuffed Portobello Mushrooms

Ingredients (continued):
- 350°F (175°C). Grease a baking dish.
- 2 cups fresh spinach leaves
- 1/2 cup crumbled feta cheese
- 2 cloves garlic, minced
- 2 tablespoons olive oil
- Salt and pepper to taste

Instructions:
1. Preheat oven to 350°F (175°C). Grease a baking dish.
2. In a skillet, heat olive oil over medium heat. Add minced garlic and sauté until fragrant.
3. Add fresh spinach leaves to the skillet and cook until wilted.
4. Remove skillet from heat and stir in crumbled feta cheese. Mix until well combined.
5. Season with salt and pepper to taste.
6. Place the portobello mushrooms in the greased baking dish, gill side up.
7. Spoon the spinach and feta mixture into the mushroom caps, dividing evenly.
8. Bake in the preheated oven for 20-25 minutes, or until the mushrooms are tender and the filling is heated through.
9. Remove from the oven and let them cool for a few minutes before serving.
10. Serve warm as a side dish or appetizer.

Nutritional Information:
- Serving Size: 1 stuffed mushroom
- Servings: 4
- Calories per serving: approximately
- Total Fat: 7g
- Carbohydrates: 5g
- Fiber: 2g
- Protein: 5g

Cooking Time:
- Prep Time: 15 minutes
- Cooking Time: 20-25 minutes

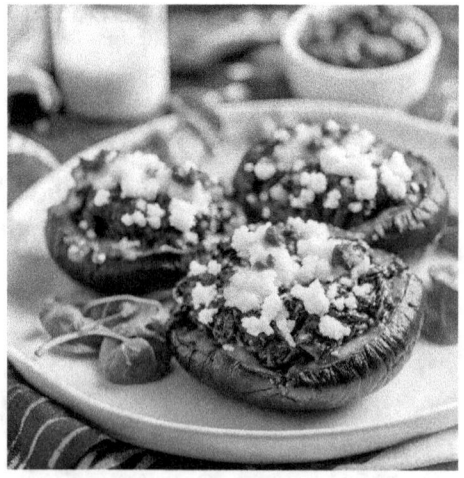

7. Mediterranean Roasted Vegetables

Ingredients:
- 2 bell peppers, sliced
- 1 small eggplant, diced
- 1 small zucchini, diced
- 1 small red onion, sliced
- 2 tomatoes, diced
- 3 cloves garlic, minced
- 2 tablespoons olive oil
- 1 teaspoon dried oregano
- 1 teaspoon dried thyme
- Salt and pepper to taste
- Fresh parsley for garnish (optional)

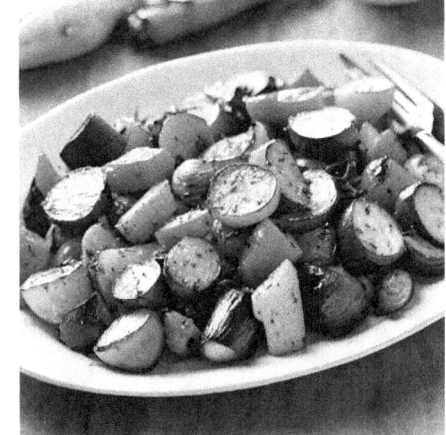

Instructions:
1. Preheat oven to 400°F (200°C). Grease a baking sheet or line with parchment paper.
2. In a large bowl, combine sliced bell peppers, diced eggplant, diced zucchini, sliced red onion, diced tomatoes, minced garlic, olive oil, dried oregano, dried thyme, salt, and pepper. Toss until vegetables are evenly coated.
3. Spread the vegetables in a single layer on the prepared baking sheet.
4. Roast in the preheated oven for 25-30 minutes, or until vegetables are tender and lightly browned, stirring halfway through.
5. Remove from the oven and transfer to a serving platter.
6. Garnish with fresh parsley if desired.
7. Serve hot or at room temperature.

Nutritional Information:
- Serving Size: 1 cup
- Servings: 4
- Calories per serving: approximately 100
- Total Fat: 7g
- Carbohydrates: 10g
- Fiber: 4g
- Protein: 2g

Cooking Time:
- Prep Time: 15 minutes
- Cooking Time: 25-30 minutes

8. Okonomiyaki

Ingredients:
- 2 cups shredded cabbage
- 1/2 cup all-purpose flour
- 2 eggs
- 1/4 cup chopped scallions
- 1/4 cup grated carrot
- 1/4 cup diced bell pepper
- 1/4 cup cooked shrimp or diced cooked chicken (optional)
- 2 tablespoons vegetable oil
- Okonomiyaki sauce or tonkatsu sauce (for serving)
- Japanese mayonnaise (for serving)
- Bonito flakes (for serving, optional)
- Aonori (dried green seaweed flakes, for serving, optional)

Instructions:
1. In a large bowl, combine shredded cabbage, all-purpose flour, eggs, chopped scallions, grated carrot, diced bell pepper, and cooked shrimp or chicken (if using). Mix until well combined.
2. Heat vegetable oil in a large skillet over medium heat.
3. Spoon the cabbage mixture into the skillet, forming individual pancakes. Flatten slightly with a spatula.
4. Cook for 3-4 minutes on each side, or until golden brown and cooked through.
5. Remove from the skillet and transfer to a serving plate.
6. Drizzle with okonomiyaki sauce or tonkatsu sauce and Japanese mayonnaise.
7. Sprinkle with bonito flakes and aonori if desired.
8. Serve hot.

Nutritional Information:
- Serving Size: 1 okonomiyaki pancake
- Servings: 4
- Calories per serving: approximately 150
- Total Fat: 8g
- Carbohydrates: 15g
- Fiber: 2g
- Protein: 6g

Cooking Time:
- Prep Time: 15 minutes
- Cooking Time: 10 minutes

9. Vietnamese Summer Rolls

Ingredients:
- 8 rice paper wrappers
- 1 cup cooked shrimp, peeled and deveined
- 1 cup rice vermicelli noodles, cooked and cooled
- 1 cup shredded lettuce
- 1 cup bean sprouts
- 1 cucumber, julienned
- 1 carrot, julienned
- Fresh mint leaves
- Fresh cilantro leaves
- Hoisin sauce (for serving)
- Peanut dipping sauce (for serving)

Instructions:
1. Fill a shallow dish with warm water. Dip one rice paper wrapper into the water for a few seconds until softened.
2. Place the softened rice paper wrapper on a clean, damp kitchen towel.
3. Arrange cooked shrimp, rice vermicelli noodles, shredded lettuce, bean sprouts, cucumber, carrot, mint leaves, and cilantro leaves in the center of the rice paper wrapper.
4. Fold the bottom of the wrapper over the filling, then fold in the sides, and roll tightly to enclose the filling.
5. Repeat with the remaining ingredients.
6. Serve the summer rolls with hoisin sauce and peanut dipping sauce on the side.

Nutritional Information:
- Serving Size: 1 summer roll
- Servings: 8
- Calories per serving: approximately 80
- Total Fat: 1g
- Carbohydrates: 15g
- Fiber: 2g
- Protein: 5g

Cooking Time:
- Prep Time: 20 minutes

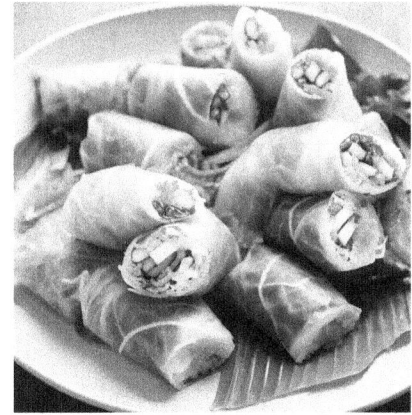

10. Ratatouille Tian

Ingredients:

- 1 eggplant, thinly sliced
- 2 zucchinis, thinly sliced
- 2 tomatoes, thinly sliced
- 1 onion, thinly sliced
- 2 cloves garlic, minced
- 2 tablespoons olive oil
- 1 tablespoon tomato paste
- 1 teaspoon dried thyme
- 1 teaspoon dried basil
- Salt and pepper to taste
- Fresh basil leaves for garnish (optional)

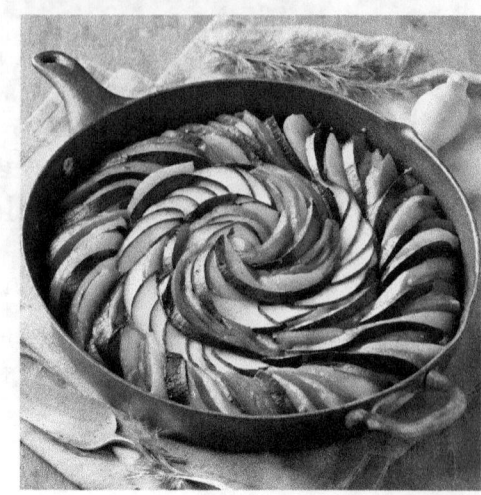

Instructions:

1. Preheat oven to 375°F (190°C). Grease a baking dish.
2. In a small bowl, mix minced garlic, olive oil, tomato paste, dried thyme, dried basil, salt, and pepper.
3. Spread a thin layer of the olive oil mixture in the bottom of the greased baking dish.
4. Arrange the sliced eggplant, zucchini, tomatoes, onion, and garlic in alternating layers in the baking dish, forming a spiral pattern.
5. Drizzle the remaining olive oil mixture over the vegetables.
6. Cover the baking dish with aluminum foil and bake in the preheated oven for 45-50 minutes, or until the vegetables are tender.
7. Remove the foil and bake for an additional 10-15 minutes, or until the top is golden brown.
8. Remove from the oven and let it cool for a few minutes before serving.
9. Garnish with fresh basil leaves if desired.
10. Serve warm as a side dish or main course.

Nutritional Information:

- Serving Size: 1/6 of the tian
- Servings: 6
- Calories per serving: approximately 100
- Total Fat: 5g Carbohydrates: 13g Fiber: 4g Protein: 3g

Cooking Time:

- Prep Time: 15 minutes   **Cooking Time**: 1 hour 5 minutes

11. Sesame Ginger Snap Peas

Ingredients:
- 1 pound snap peas, trimmed
- 2 tablespoons soy sauce
- 1 tablespoon rice vinegar
- 1 tablespoon honey or maple syrup
- 1 teaspoon sesame oil
- 1 teaspoon grated ginger
- 2 cloves garlic, minced
- 1 tablespoon vegetable oil
- 1 tablespoon sesame seeds
- Salt and pepper to taste

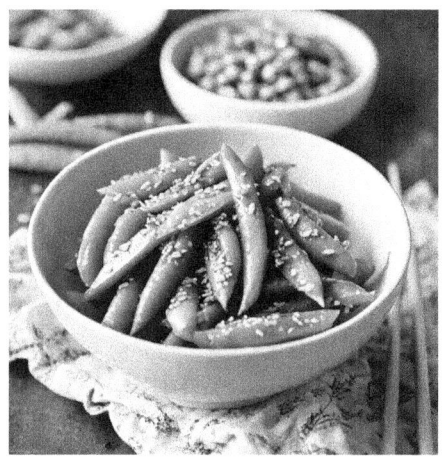

Instructions:
1. In a small bowl, whisk together soy sauce, rice vinegar, honey or maple syrup, sesame oil, grated ginger, and minced garlic to make the sauce.
2. Heat vegetable oil in a skillet or wok over high heat.
3. Add snap peas to the skillet and stir-fry for 2-3 minutes until slightly tender but still crisp.
4. Pour the sauce over the snap peas and toss to coat evenly.
5. Cook for another 1-2 minutes until the sauce thickens slightly.
6. Remove from heat and sprinkle sesame seeds on top.
7. Season with salt and pepper to taste.
8. Serve hot as a side dish.

Nutritional Information:
- Serving Size: 1/2 cup
- Servings: 4
- Calories per serving: approximately 70
- Total Fat: 3g
- Carbohydrates: 9g
- Fiber: 2g
- Protein: 2g

Cooking Time:
- Prep Time: 10 minutes
- Cooking Time: 5 minutes

12. Stuffed Mushrooms

Ingredients:
- 12 large mushrooms, stems removed and reserved
- 1/2 cup breadcrumbs
- 1/4 cup grated Parmesan cheese
- 2 tablespoons chopped fresh parsley
- 2 cloves garlic, minced
- 2 tablespoons olive oil
- Salt and pepper to taste

Instructions:
1. Preheat oven to 375°F (190°C). Grease a baking dish.
2. In a mixing bowl, combine chopped mushroom stems, breadcrumbs, grated Parmesan cheese, chopped fresh parsley, minced garlic, olive oil, salt, and pepper. Mix until well combined.
3. Spoon the filling into the mushroom caps, pressing gently to pack the filling.
4. Place the stuffed mushrooms in the greased baking dish.
5. Bake in the preheated oven for 20-25 minutes, or until the mushrooms are tender and the filling is golden brown.
6. Remove from the oven and let them cool for a few minutes before serving.
7. Serve warm as an appetizer or side dish.

Nutritional Information:
- Serving Size: 2 stuffed mushrooms
- Servings: 6
- Calories per serving: approximately 90
- Total Fat: 5g
- Carbohydrates: 8g
- Fiber: 1g
- Protein: 4g

Cooking Time:
- Prep Time: 15 minutes
- Cooking Time: 20-25 minutes

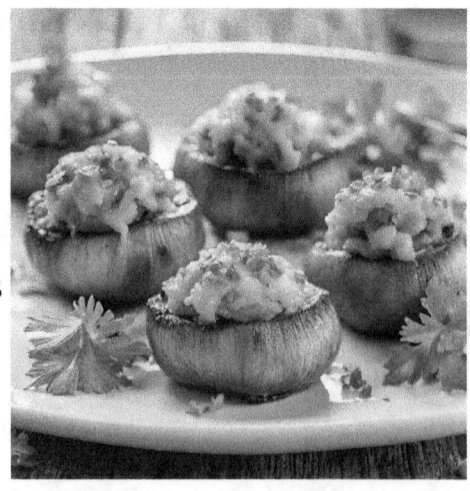

13. Vegetable Paella

Ingredients:
- 1 tablespoon olive oil
- 1 onion, diced
- 2 cloves garlic, minced
- 1 red bell pepper, diced
- 1 yellow bell pepper, diced
- 1 cup diced tomatoes (canned or fresh)
- 1 teaspoon smoked paprika
- 1/2 teaspoon saffron threads
- 1 cup Arborio rice
- 2 cups vegetable broth
- 1 cup frozen peas
- Salt and pepper to taste
- Lemon wedges for serving
- Chopped fresh parsley for garnish (optional)

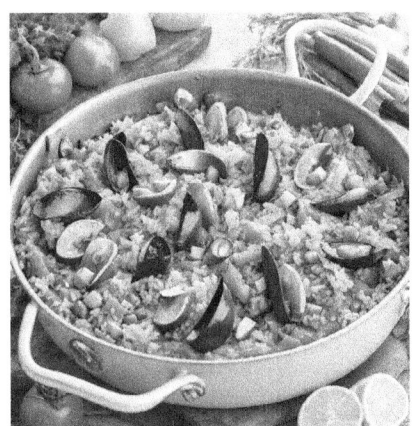

Instructions:
1. In a large skillet or paella pan, heat olive oil over medium heat.
2. Add diced onion and minced garlic to the skillet. Sauté until softened and fragrant.
3. Add diced red bell pepper and yellow bell pepper to the skillet. Cook until slightly softened.
4. Stir in diced tomatoes, smoked paprika, and saffron threads. Cook for 2-3 minutes.
5. Add Arborio rice to the skillet and stir to coat with the vegetable mixture.
6. Pour vegetable broth into the skillet and bring to a simmer.
7. Reduce heat to low, cover, and cook for 15-20 minutes, or until the rice is tender and most of the liquid has been absorbed.
8. Stir in frozen peas and cook for another 2-3 minutes until heated through.
9. Season with salt and pepper to taste.
10. Remove from heat and let it rest for a few minutes.
11. Garnish with chopped fresh parsley if desired.
12. Serve hot with lemon wedges on the side.

Nutritional Information:

Servings: 4 Calories per serving: approximately 250
- Total Fat: 4g Carbohydrates: 49g Fiber: 5g Protein: 6g

Cooking Time: 30-35 minutes

14. Zucchini Noodles with Pesto

Ingredients:
- 4 medium zucchinis
- 1 cup fresh basil leaves
- 1/4 cup pine nuts
- 2 cloves garlic
- 1/4 cup grated Parmesan cheese
- 1/4 cup olive oil
- Salt and pepper to taste
- Cherry tomatoes for garnish (optional)

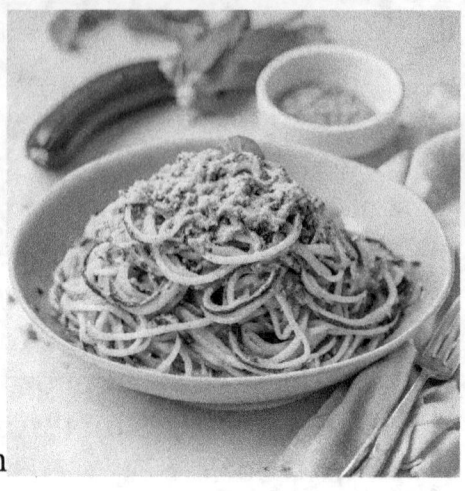

Instructions:
1. Using a spiralizer, spiralize the zucchinis to make zucchini noodles.
2. In a food processor, combine fresh basil leaves, pine nuts, garlic, and grated Parmesan cheese. Pulse until finely chopped.
3. With the food processor running, gradually add olive oil until the pesto reaches a smooth consistency.
4. Season the pesto with salt and pepper to taste.
5. In a large skillet, heat olive oil over medium heat. Add zucchini noodles and sauté for 2-3 minutes until heated through.
6. Add the pesto to the skillet and toss to coat the zucchini noodles evenly.
7. Cook for another 1-2 minutes until the pesto is warmed.
8. Remove from heat and transfer to serving plates.
9. Garnish with cherry tomatoes if desired.
10. Serve immediately.

Nutritional Information:
- Serving Size: 1 cup
- Servings: 4
- Calories per serving: approximately 200
- Total Fat: 17g
- Carbohydrates: 8g
- Fiber: 2g
- Protein: 5g

Cooking Time:
- Prep Time: 15 minutes
- Cooking Time: 5 minutes

15. Thai Green Papaya Salad

Ingredients:
- 1 green papaya, peeled and julienned
- 1 carrot, peeled and julienned
- 1/2 cup cherry tomatoes, halved
- 1/4 cup chopped peanuts
- 2 tablespoons fish sauce
- 2 tablespoons lime juice
- 1 tablespoon palm sugar or brown sugar
- 1-2 Thai bird's eye chilies, thinly sliced (optional)
- 2 cloves garlic, minced
- 2 tablespoons dried shrimp, soaked in water (optional)
- Fresh cilantro leaves for garnish
- Fresh mint leaves for garnish

Instructions:
1. In a large bowl, combine julienned green papaya, julienned carrot, cherry tomatoes, chopped peanuts, fish sauce, lime juice, palm sugar or brown sugar, thinly sliced Thai bird's eye chilies (if using), minced garlic, and soaked dried shrimp (if using). Toss until well combined.
2. Taste and adjust seasoning if needed.
3. Transfer the salad to a serving plate.
4. Garnish with fresh cilantro leaves and mint leaves.
5. Serve immediately as a refreshing appetizer or side dish.

Nutritional Information:
- Serving Size: 1 cup
- Servings: 4
- Calories per serving: approximately 120
- Total Fat: 7g
- Carbohydrates: 12g
- Fiber: 3g
- Protein: 5g

Cooking Time:
- Prep Time: 20 minutes

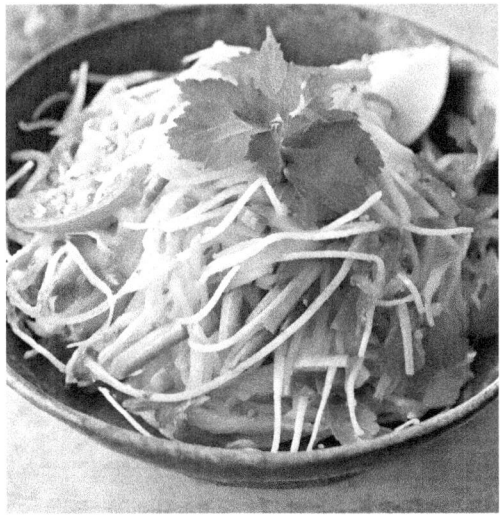

16. Miso Glazed Eggplant

Ingredients:
- 2 large eggplants, sliced lengthwise
- 2 tablespoons white miso paste
- 2 tablespoons mirin
- 1 tablespoon soy sauce
- 1 tablespoon honey or maple syrup
- 1 tablespoon rice vinegar
- 1 teaspoon sesame oil
- 2 cloves garlic, minced
- 1 tablespoon grated ginger
- Toasted sesame seeds for garnish
- Sliced green onions for garnish

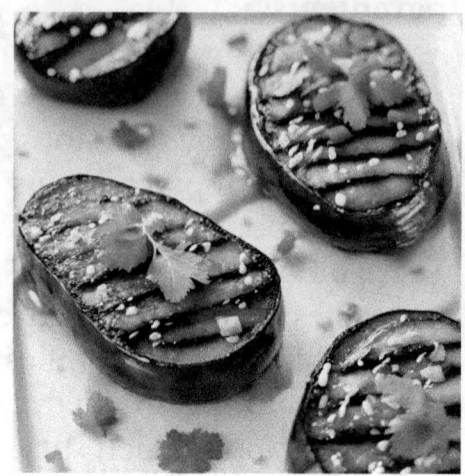

Instructions:
1. Preheat oven to 400°F (200°C). Grease a baking dish.
2. In a small bowl, whisk together white miso paste, mirin, soy sauce, honey or maple syrup, rice vinegar, sesame oil, minced garlic, and grated ginger to make the glaze.
3. Place the sliced eggplants in a single layer in the greased baking dish.
4. Brush the miso glaze over the eggplant slices, coating them evenly.
5. Bake in the preheated oven for 20-25 minutes, or until the eggplants are tender and caramelized, brushing with additional glaze halfway through.
6. Remove from the oven and let them cool for a few minutes.
7. Transfer to a serving plate and garnish with toasted sesame seeds and sliced green onions.
8. Serve hot as a flavorful side dish or appetizer.

Nutritional Information:
- Serving Size: 1/2 eggplant
- Servings: 4
- Calories per serving: approximately 120
- Total Fat: 3g
- Carbohydrates: 22g   Fiber: 7g
- Protein: 4g

Cooking Time:
- Prep Time: 15 minutes
- Cooking Time: 20-25 minutes

17. Italian Marinated Grilled Vegetables

Ingredients:
- 2 zucchinis, sliced lengthwise
- 2 yellow squash, sliced lengthwise
- 1 eggplant, sliced
- 1 red bell pepper, seeded and sliced
- 1 yellow bell pepper, seeded and sliced
- 1/4 cup olive oil
- 2 tablespoons balsamic vinegar
- 2 cloves garlic, minced
- 1 teaspoon dried oregano
- 1 teaspoon dried basil
- Salt and pepper to taste
- Fresh basil leaves for garnish (optional)

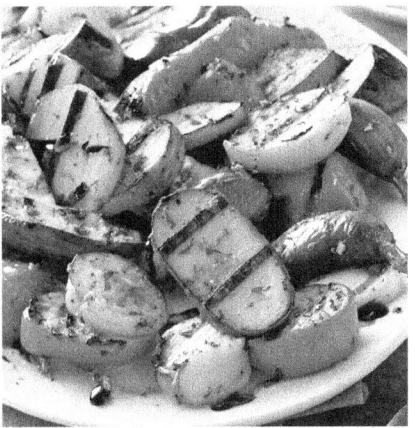

Instructions:
1. In a small bowl, whisk together olive oil, balsamic vinegar, minced garlic, dried oregano, dried basil, salt, and pepper to make the marinade.
2. Place sliced zucchinis, yellow squash, eggplant, red bell pepper, and yellow bell pepper in a large shallow dish. Pour the marinade over the vegetables and toss to coat evenly.
3. Cover and refrigerate for at least 30 minutes to marinate.
4. Preheat grill to medium-high heat.
5. Remove the vegetables from the marinade and place them on the grill.
6. Grill for 4-5 minutes per side, or until tender and lightly charred.
7. Remove from the grill and transfer to a serving platter.
8. Garnish with fresh basil leaves if desired.
9. Serve hot or at room temperature.

Nutritional Information:
- Serving Size: 1 cup
- Servings: 4
- Calories per serving: approximately 120
- Total Fat: 7g Carbohydrates: 14g Fiber: 5g   Protein: 3g

Cooking Time:
- Prep Time: 10 minutes
- Marinating Time: 30 minutes
- Cooking Time: 10-12 minutes

18. Vegetable Spring Rolls

Ingredients:
- 8 spring roll wrappers
- 2 cups mixed shredded vegetables (such as carrots, cabbage, bell peppers, cucumber)
- 1/2 cup cooked rice vermicelli noodles
- Fresh herbs (such as mint leaves, cilantro leaves)
- 1/4 cup hoisin sauce
- 1/4 cup peanut dipping sauce

Instructions:
1. Prepare a shallow dish with warm water.
2. Dip one spring roll wrapper into the water for a few seconds until softened.
3. Place the softened wrapper on a clean, damp kitchen towel.
4. Arrange shredded vegetables, rice vermicelli noodles, and fresh herbs in the center of the wrapper.
5. Fold the bottom of the wrapper over the filling, then fold in the sides, and roll tightly to enclose the filling.
6. Repeat with the remaining wrappers and filling.
7. Serve the spring rolls with hoisin sauce and peanut dipping sauce on the side.

Nutritional Information:
- Serving Size: 1 spring roll
- Servings: 8
- Calories per serving: approximately 80
- Total Fat: 1g
- Carbohydrates: 16g
- Fiber: 2g
- Protein: 2g

Cooking Time:
- Prep Time: 20 minutes

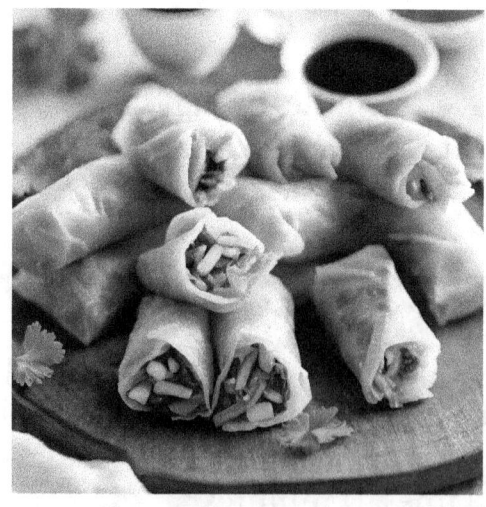

19. Cucumber Salad

Ingredients:
- 2 English cucumbers, thinly sliced
- 1/4 cup rice vinegar
- 1 tablespoon sesame oil
- 1 tablespoon soy sauce
- 1 teaspoon honey or maple syrup
- 1 teaspoon grated ginger
- 1 clove garlic, minced
- 1 tablespoon toasted sesame seeds
- 2 green onions, thinly sliced
- Salt and pepper to taste

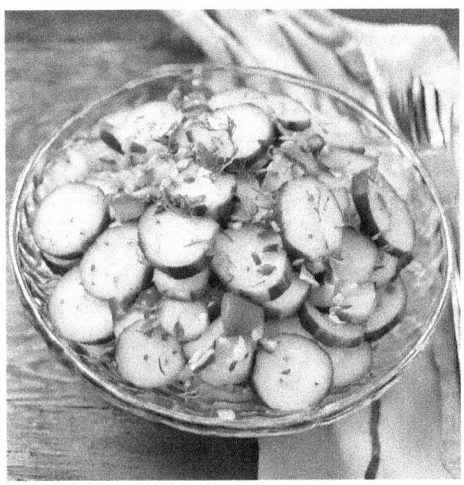

Instructions:
1. In a large bowl, whisk together rice vinegar, sesame oil, soy sauce, honey or maple syrup, grated ginger, minced garlic, salt, and pepper to make the dressing.
2. Add thinly sliced cucumbers to the bowl and toss to coat with the dressing.
3. Let the cucumber salad marinate in the refrigerator for at least 30 minutes.
4. Before serving, sprinkle toasted sesame seeds and thinly sliced green onions on top.
5. Serve chilled as a refreshing side dish.

Nutritional Information:
- Serving Size: 1 cup
- Servings: 4
- Calories per serving: approximately 50
- Total Fat: 2g
- Carbohydrates: 7g
- Fiber: 1g
- Protein: 1g

Cooking Time:
- Prep Time: 10 minutes
- Marinating Time: 30 minutes

20. Vegetable Curry

Ingredients:
- 2 tablespoons coconut oil
- 1 onion, diced
- 2 cloves garlic, minced
- 1 tablespoon grated ginger
- 2 carrots, peeled and diced
- 1 bell pepper, diced
- 1 zucchini, diced
- 1 cup cauliflower florets
- 1 cup green beans, trimmed and cut into bite-sized pieces
- 1 can (14 oz) coconut milk
- 2 tablespoons red curry paste
- 1 tablespoon soy sauce
- 1 tablespoon maple syrup or brown sugar
- Salt and pepper to taste
- Fresh cilantro for garnish (optional)
- Cooked rice for serving

Instructions:
1. In a large skillet or pot, heat coconut oil over medium heat.
2. Add diced onion, minced garlic, and grated ginger to the skillet. Sauté until softened and fragrant.
3. Stir in diced carrots, bell pepper, zucchini, cauliflower florets, and green beans. Cook for 5-7 minutes until the vegetables are slightly tender.
4. In a small bowl, whisk together coconut milk, red curry paste, soy sauce, maple syrup or brown sugar, salt, and pepper.
5. Pour the curry sauce over the vegetables in the skillet. Stir to combine.
6. Bring the mixture to a simmer and cook for 10-12 minutes, stirring occasionally, until the vegetables are cooked through and the sauce has thickened.
7. Taste and adjust seasoning if necessary.
8. Remove from heat and let it cool slightly.
9. Garnish with fresh cilantro if desired.
10. Serve the vegetable curry hot over cooked rice.

Nutritional Information:
- Serving Size: 1 cup curry with rice
- Servings: 4
- Calories per serving: approximately 300
- Total Fat: 20g
- Carbohydrates: 30g
- Fiber: 6g
- Protein: 5g

Cooking Time:
- Prep Time: 15 minutes
- Cooking Time: 25 minutes

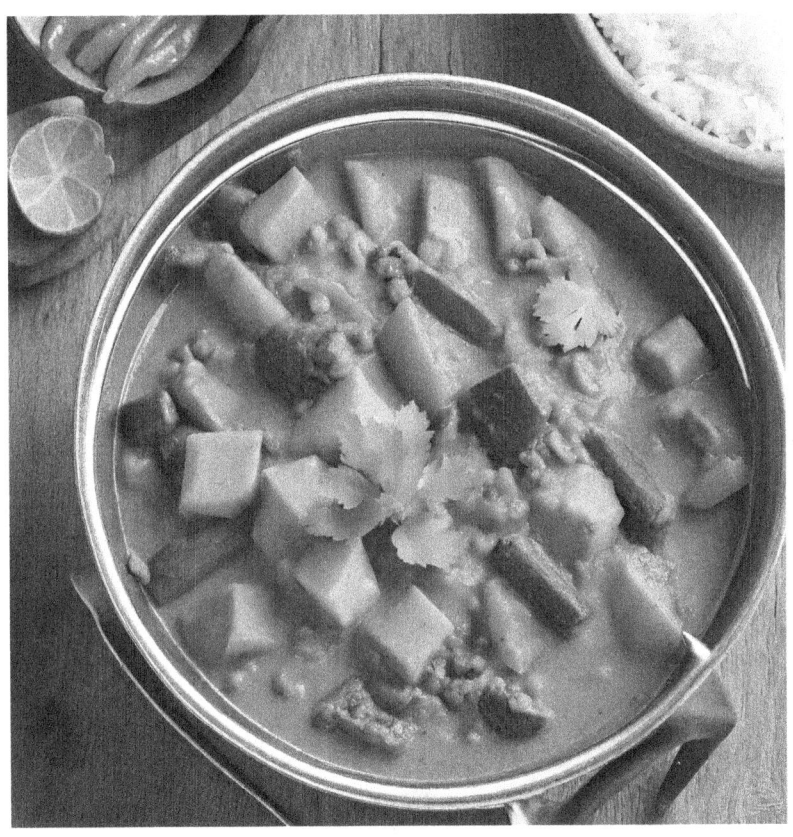

21. Caprese Salad

Ingredients:
- 2 large ripe tomatoes, sliced
- 1 pound fresh mozzarella cheese, sliced
- Fresh basil leaves
- Balsamic glaze (optional)
- Extra virgin olive oil
- Salt and pepper to taste

Instructions:
1. Arrange alternating slices of tomatoes, mozzarella cheese, and fresh basil leaves on a serving platter.
2. Drizzle with balsamic glaze (if using) and extra virgin olive oil.
3. Season with salt and pepper to taste.
4. Serve immediately as a refreshing salad.

Nutritional Information:
- Serving Size: 1/4 of the salad
- Servings: 4
- Calories per serving: approximately 250
- Total Fat: 20g
- Carbohydrates: 5g
- Fiber: 1g
- Protein: 15g

Cooking Time:
- Prep Time: 10 minutes

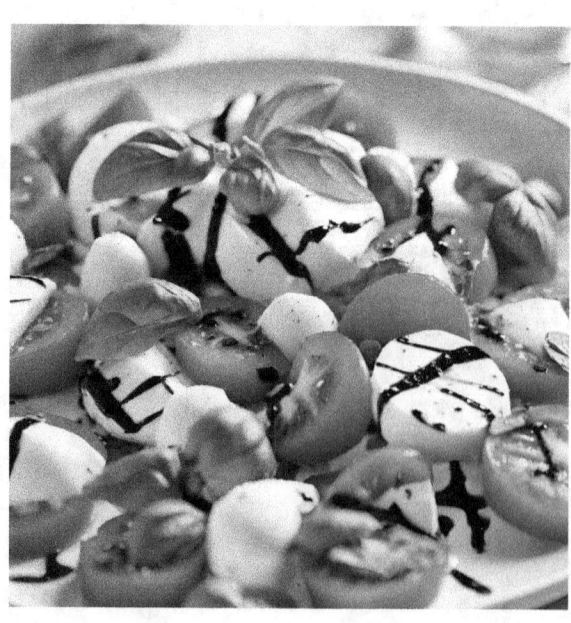

22. Greek Salad

Ingredients:
- 2 large tomatoes, diced
- 1 cucumber, diced
- 1/2 red onion, thinly sliced
- 1/2 cup Kalamata olives
- 1/2 cup crumbled feta cheese
- 2 tablespoons extra virgin olive oil
- 1 tablespoon red wine vinegar
- 1 teaspoon dried oregano
- Salt and pepper to taste

Instructions:
1. In a large bowl, combine diced tomatoes, diced cucumber, thinly sliced red onion, Kalamata olives, and crumbled feta cheese.
2. In a small bowl, whisk together extra virgin olive oil, red wine vinegar, dried oregano, salt, and pepper to make the dressing.
3. Pour the dressing over the salad and toss to coat evenly.
4. Serve immediately as a flavorful side dish or appetizer.

Nutritional Information:
- Serving Size: 1 cup
- Servings: 4
- Calories per serving: approximately 150
- Total Fat: 12g
- Carbohydrates: 8g
- Fiber: 2g
- Protein: 4g

Cooking Time:
- Prep Time: 10 minutes

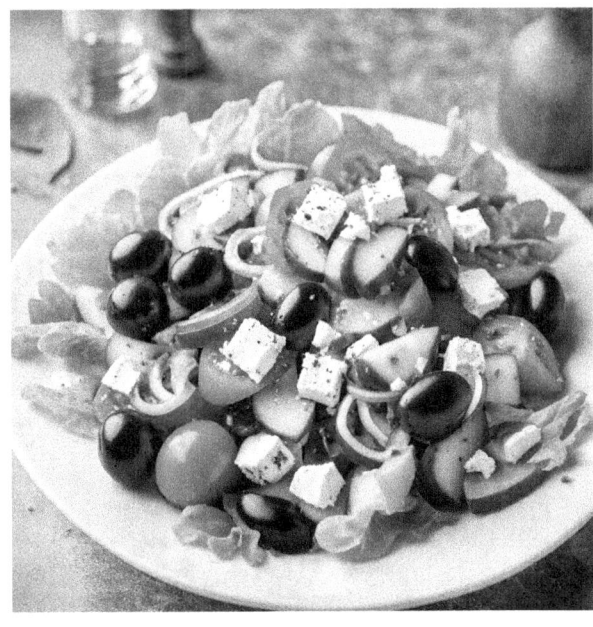

23. Stuffed Bell Peppers

Ingredients:
- 4 large bell peppers (any color), halved and seeded
- 1 cup cooked quinoa or rice
- 1 cup cooked black beans
- 1 cup corn kernels (fresh, canned, or frozen)
- 1 cup diced tomatoes
- 1/2 cup diced onion
- 2 cloves garlic, minced
- 1 teaspoon ground cumin
- 1 teaspoon chili powder
- Salt and pepper to taste
- 1/2 cup shredded cheddar cheese (optional)
- Fresh cilantro for garnish (optional)

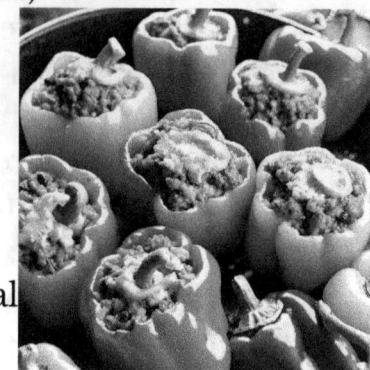

Instructions:
1. Preheat oven to 375°F (190°C). Grease a baking dish.
2. Place halved bell peppers in the greased baking dish, cut side up.
3. In a large bowl, combine cooked quinoa or rice, cooked black beans, corn kernels, diced tomatoes, diced onion, minced garlic, ground cumin, chili powder, salt, and pepper. Mix until well combined.
4. Spoon the quinoa mixture into each bell pepper half, pressing gently to pack the filling.
5. Cover the baking dish with aluminum foil and bake in the preheated oven for 30-35 minutes, or until the peppers are tender.
6. If using shredded cheddar cheese, remove the foil, sprinkle cheese over the stuffed peppers, and bake for an additional 5 minutes until the cheese is melted and bubbly.
7. Remove from the oven and let them cool for a few minutes.
8. Garnish with fresh cilantro if desired.
9. Serve warm as a satisfying main dish.

Nutritional Information:
- Serving Size: 1 stuffed bell pepper half
- Servings: 8
- Calories per serving: approximately 150
- Total Fat: 3g   Carbohydrates: 25g   Fiber: 6g   Protein: 7g

Cooking Time:
- Prep Time: 20 minutes   Cooking Time: 35-40 minutes

POULTRY AND MEAT

1. American BBQ Chicken Drumsticks
Ingredients:
- 8 chicken drumsticks
- 1 cup BBQ sauce
- 2 tablespoons olive oil
- 1 teaspoon garlic powder
- 1 teaspoon onion powder
- Salt and pepper to taste
- Chopped fresh parsley for garnish (optional)

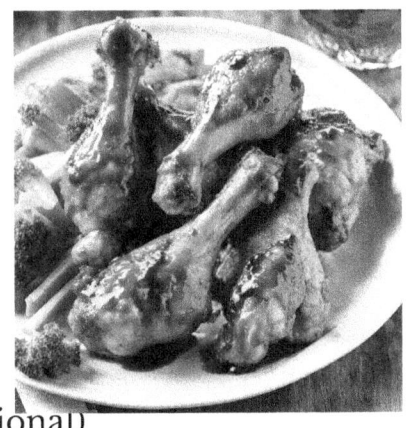

Instructions:
1. Preheat the grill to medium-high heat.
2. In a small bowl, mix together BBQ sauce, olive oil, garlic powder, onion powder, salt, and pepper to make the marinade.
3. Pat the chicken drumsticks dry with paper towels and place them in a large bowl.
4. Pour the marinade over the chicken drumsticks and toss to coat evenly.
5. Let the chicken marinate for at least 30 minutes, or up to 4 hours in the refrigerator.
6. Remove the chicken from the marinade and grill for 25-30 minutes, turning occasionally, until cooked through and the internal temperature reaches 165°F (74°C).
7. Remove from the grill and let them rest for a few minutes.
8. Garnish with chopped fresh parsley if desired.
9. Serve hot.

Nutritional Information:
- Serving Size: 1 drumstick
- Servings: 8
- Calories per serving: approximately 200
- Total Fat: 8g
- Carbohydrates: 12g Fiber: 1g Protein: 18g

Cooking Time:
- Prep Time: 10 minutes
- Marinating Time: 30 minutes to 4 hours
- Cooking Time: 25-30 minutes

2. German Sauerbraten

Ingredients:
- 2 pounds beef roast (such as chuck or round)
- 1 onion, sliced
- 2 carrots, sliced
- 2 celery stalks, sliced
- 2 cups beef broth
- 1 cup red wine vinegar
- 1/2 cup water
- 1/4 cup brown sugar
- 2 tablespoons whole grain mustard
- 2 tablespoons pickling spices (such as peppercorns, cloves, allspice, bay leaves)
- 2 tablespoons vegetable oil
- Salt and pepper to taste
- Chopped fresh parsley for garnish (optional)

Instructions:
1. In a large bowl, combine beef broth, red wine vinegar, water, brown sugar, whole grain mustard, and pickling spices. Mix until the sugar is dissolved.
2. Place the beef roast in a resealable plastic bag or a glass dish. Pour the marinade over the beef roast, making sure it is fully submerged. Marinate in the refrigerator for 2-3 days, turning occasionally.
3. After marinating, remove the beef roast from the marinade and pat dry with paper towels. Reserve the marinade.
4. Preheat the oven to 325°F (160°C).
5. Heat vegetable oil in a Dutch oven or large oven-safe pot over medium-high heat.
6. Sear the beef roast on all sides until browned, about 8-10 minutes.
7. Add sliced onion, carrots, and celery to the pot. Cook for 5 minutes until softened.
8. Pour the reserved marinade over the beef roast and vegetables.
9. Cover the pot and transfer to the preheated oven.
10. Bake for 3-4 hours, or until the beef is tender and can be easily shredded with a fork.
11. Remove from the oven and let it rest for a few minutes.
12. Garnish with chopped fresh parsley if desired.

Nutritional Information:
- Serving Size: 1/8 of the recipe
- Servings: 8
- Calories per serving: approximately 350
- Total Fat: 15g
- Carbohydrates: 10g
- Fiber: 1g
- Protein: 35g

Cooking Time:
- Prep Time: 15 minutes
- Marinating Time: 2-3 days
- Cooking Time: 3-4 hours

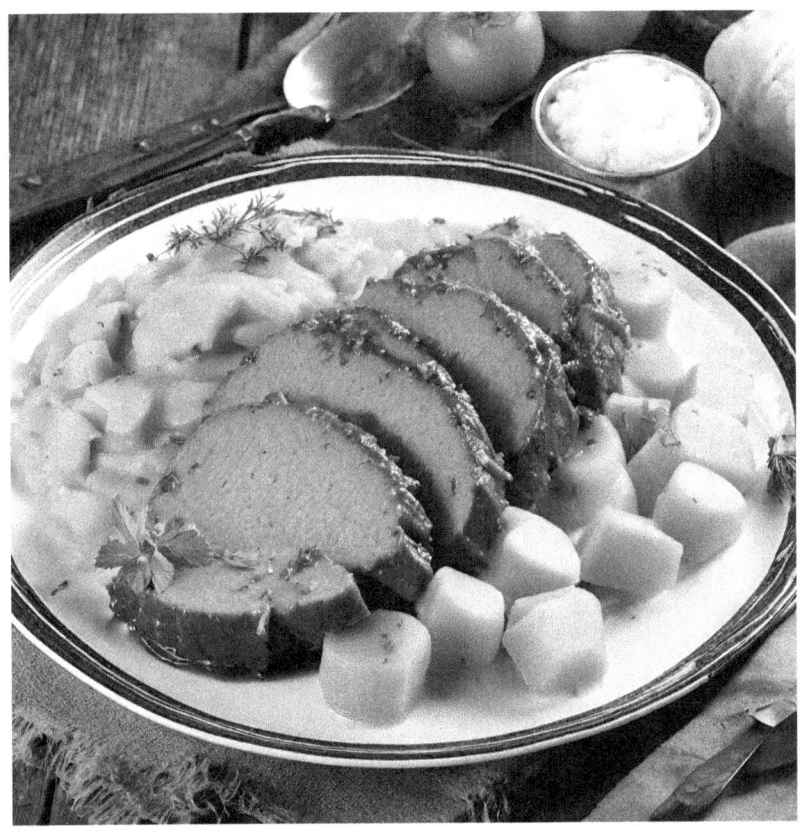

3. Thai Basil Beef

Ingredients:
- 1 pound beef sirloin, thinly sliced
- 2 tablespoons vegetable oil
- 3 cloves garlic, minced
- 2 Thai bird's eye chilies, thinly sliced
- 1 onion, thinly sliced
- 1 bell pepper, thinly sliced
- 1 cup fresh basil leaves
- 2 tablespoons soy sauce
- 1 tablespoon fish sauce
- 1 tablespoon oyster sauce
- 1 teaspoon sugar
- Cooked rice for serving

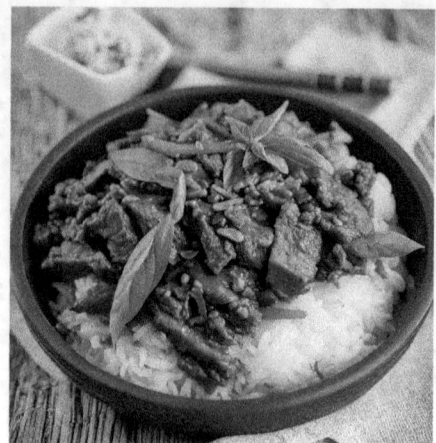

Instructions:
1. Heat vegetable oil in a wok or large skillet over high heat.
2. Add minced garlic and sliced Thai bird's eye chilies to the wok. Stir-fry for 30 seconds until fragrant.
3. Add thinly sliced beef sirloin to the wok. Stir-fry for 2-3 minutes until browned.
4. Add thinly sliced onion and bell pepper to the wok. Stir-fry for another 2-3 minutes until the vegetables are tender-crisp.
5. Stir in soy sauce, fish sauce, oyster sauce, and sugar. Cook for an additional minute, stirring constantly.
6. Remove the wok from the heat and stir in fresh basil leaves until wilted.
7. Serve the Thai basil beef hot over cooked rice.

Nutritional Information:
- Serving Size: 1/4 of the recipe (excluding rice)
- Servings: 4
- Calories per serving: approximately 250
- Total Fat: 12g
- Carbohydrates: 7g
- Fiber: 2g
- Protein: 28g

Cooking Time:
- Prep Time: 15 minutes
- Cooking Time: 10 minutes

4. Mexican Chicken Tinga Tacos
Ingredients:
- 1 pound boneless, skinless chicken breasts
- 1 onion, chopped
- 2 cloves garlic, minced
- 1 can (14 oz) diced tomatoes
- 2 chipotle peppers in adobo sauce, chopped
- 1 teaspoon dried oregano
- 1 teaspoon ground cumin
- Salt and pepper to taste
- Corn or flour tortillas
- Toppings: diced avocado, chopped cilantro, lime wedges

Instructions:
1. In a large skillet or pot, combine chopped onion, minced garlic, diced tomatoes, chipotle peppers in adobo sauce, dried oregano, ground cumin, salt, and pepper.
2. Place chicken breasts on top of the tomato mixture.
3. Cover and simmer over medium heat for 20-25 minutes, or until the chicken is cooked through and tender.
4. Remove the chicken from the skillet and shred using two forks.
5. Return the shredded chicken to the skillet and stir to combine with the tomato mixture.
6. Cook for an additional 5 minutes to allow the flavors to meld.
7. Warm the tortillas according to package instructions.
8. Spoon the chicken tinga mixture onto the warm tortillas.
9. Serve tacos topped with diced avocado, chopped cilantro, and lime wedges.

Nutritional Information:
- Serving Size: 2 tacos
- Servings: 4
- Calories per serving: approximately 300
- Total Fat: 8g
- Carbohydrates: 25g
- Fiber: 5g
- Protein: 30g

Cooking Time:
- Prep Time: 10 minutes
- Cooking Time: 30-35 minutes

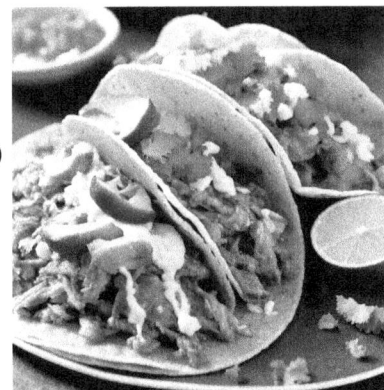

5. Japanese Yakitori Skewers

Ingredients:
- 1 pound boneless, skinless chicken thighs, cut into bite-sized pieces
- 1/4 cup soy sauce
- 2 tablespoons sake (or dry white wine)
- 2 tablespoons mirin
- 1 tablespoon brown sugar
- 1 clove garlic, minced
- 1 teaspoon grated ginger
- Bamboo skewers, soaked in water

Instructions:
1. In a bowl, whisk together soy sauce, sake, mirin, brown sugar, minced garlic, and grated ginger to make the marinade.
2. Add chicken thigh pieces to the marinade and toss to coat evenly. Let marinate for at least 30 minutes in the refrigerator.
3. Preheat grill or grill pan over medium-high heat.
4. Thread marinated chicken pieces onto soaked bamboo skewers.
5. Grill the yakitori skewers for 5-6 minutes on each side, or until cooked through and slightly charred.
6. Remove from the grill and let them rest for a few minutes.
7. Serve hot as a delicious appetizer or main dish.

Nutritional Information:
- Serving Size: 2 skewers
- Servings: 4
- Calories per serving: approximately 200
- Total Fat: 8g
- Carbohydrates: 6g
- Fiber: 0g
- Protein: 25g

Cooking Time:
- Prep Time: 10 minutes
- Marinating Time: 30 minutes
- Cooking Time: 12-15 minutes

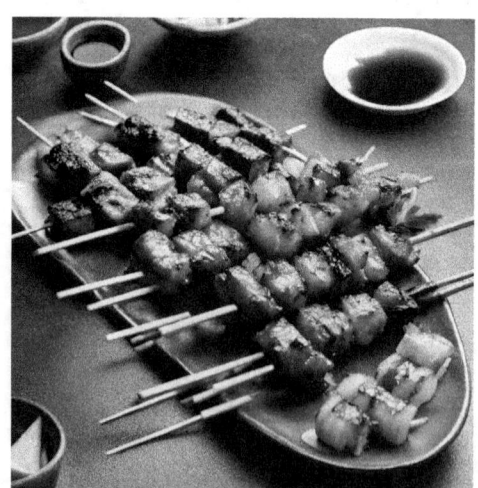

6. Brazilian Feijoada

Ingredients:
- 1 lb black beans, soaked overnight
- 1 lb pork shoulder, diced
- 1 lb beef ribs
- 1 lb smoked sausage, sliced
- 1 onion, chopped
- 4 cloves garlic, minced
- 2 bay leaves
- Salt and pepper to taste
- Cooked rice for serving
- Orange slices for garnish (optional)

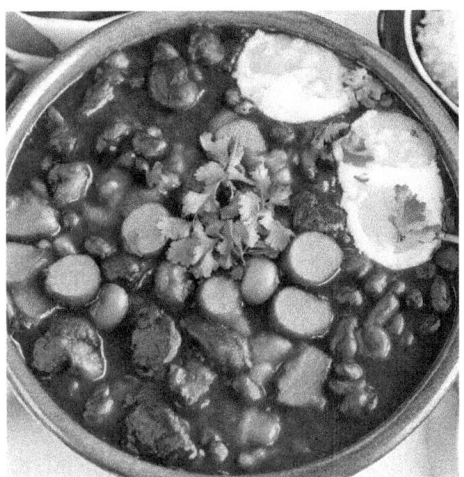

Instructions:
1. In a large pot, combine soaked black beans, diced pork shoulder, beef ribs, sliced smoked sausage, chopped onion, minced garlic, and bay leaves.
2. Add enough water to cover the ingredients and bring to a boil.
3. Reduce heat to low, cover, and simmer for 2-3 hours, or until the beans and meat are tender, stirring occasionally.
4. Season with salt and pepper to taste.
5. Serve the feijoada hot over cooked rice.
6. Garnish with orange slices if desired.

Nutritional Information:
- Serving Size: 1 cup feijoada with rice
- Servings: 8
- Calories per serving: approximately 400
- Total Fat: 18g
- Carbohydrates: 38g
- Fiber: 10g
- Protein: 24g

Cooking Time:
- Prep Time: 15 minutes (plus overnight soaking)
- Cooking Time: 2-3 hours

7. Swedish Meatballs

Ingredients:
- 1 lb ground beef
- 1/2 lb ground pork
- 1/2 cup breadcrumbs
- 1/4 cup milk
- 1 egg
- 1 onion, finely chopped
- 2 cloves garlic, minced
- 1 teaspoon salt
- 1/2 teaspoon black pepper
- 1/4 teaspoon ground nutmeg
- 1/4 teaspoon ground allspice
- 2 tablespoons butter
- 2 tablespoons all-purpose flour
- 2 cups beef broth
- 1/2 cup sour cream
- Chopped fresh parsley for garnish (optional)

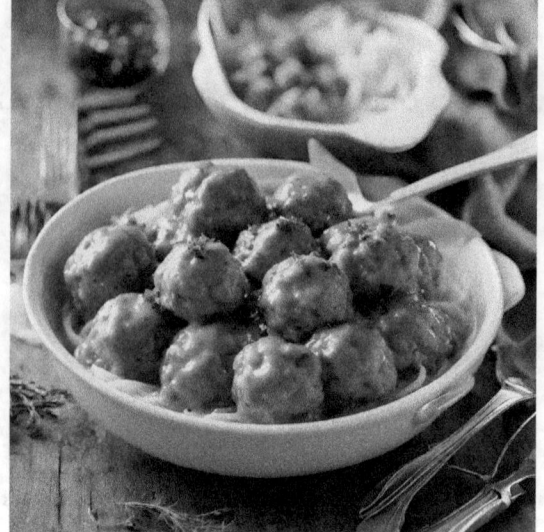

Instructions:
1. In a large bowl, combine ground beef, ground pork, breadcrumbs, milk, egg, chopped onion, minced garlic, salt, black pepper, nutmeg, and allspice. Mix until well combined.
2. Shape the mixture into small meatballs.
3. In a large skillet, melt butter over medium heat. Add the meatballs and cook until browned on all sides, about 8-10 minutes.
4. Remove the meatballs from the skillet and set aside.
5. In the same skillet, whisk in flour and cook for 1-2 minutes.
6. Gradually whisk in beef broth until smooth.
7. Return the meatballs to the skillet and simmer in the gravy for 10-15 minutes, or until cooked through.
8. Stir in sour cream and cook for an additional 2-3 minutes.
9. Garnish with chopped fresh parsley if desired.
10. Serve the Swedish meatballs hot with mashed potatoes or noodles.

Nutritional Information:

Servings: 6   Calories per serving: approximately 350
- Total Fat: 22g Carbohydrates: 12g Fiber: 1g Protein: 25g

Cooking Time: 30 minutes

8. Lebanese Grilled Chicken Shawarma

Ingredients:
- 1 lb boneless, skinless chicken thighs
- 1/4 cup plain yogurt
- 2 tablespoons olive oil
- 2 cloves garlic, minced
- 1 teaspoon ground cumin
- 1 teaspoon paprika
- 1/2 teaspoon ground turmeric
- 1/2 teaspoon ground cinnamon
- 1/4 teaspoon cayenne pepper
- Salt and pepper to taste
- Pita bread, for serving
- Toppings: chopped tomatoes, cucumbers, onions, tahini sauce

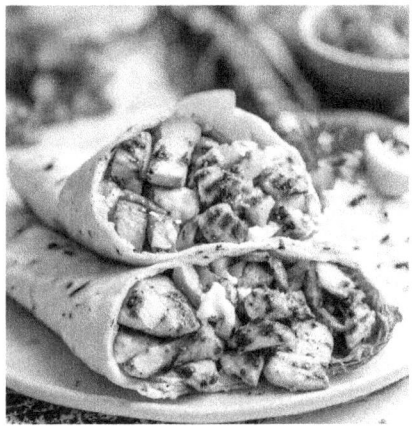

Instructions:
1. In a bowl, combine plain yogurt, olive oil, minced garlic, ground cumin, paprika, ground turmeric, ground cinnamon, cayenne pepper, salt, and pepper to make the marinade.
2. Add chicken thighs to the marinade and toss to coat evenly. Let marinate in the refrigerator for at least 1 hour, or overnight for best flavor.
3. Preheat grill to medium-high heat.
4. Remove the chicken thighs from the marinade and shake off any excess.
5. Grill the chicken thighs for 6-8 minutes per side, or until cooked through and charred.
6. Remove from the grill and let them rest for a few minutes.
7. Slice the grilled chicken thighs thinly.
8. Serve the Lebanese chicken shawarma hot wrapped in pita bread with chopped tomatoes, cucumbers, onions, and tahini sauce.

Nutritional Information:
- Serving Size: 1 chicken thigh (about 4 oz)
- Servings: 4
- Calories per serving: approximately 200   Total Fat: 10g
- Carbohydrates: 2g Fiber: 0g Protein: 25g

Cooking Time:
- Prep Time: 10 minutes (plus marinating time)
- Cooking Time: 15 minutes

9. Asian Orange Glazed Duck Breast

Ingredients:
- 4 duck breasts
- Salt and pepper to taste
- 1/2 cup orange juice
- 1/4 cup soy sauce
- 2 tablespoons honey
- 2 cloves garlic, minced
- 1 teaspoon grated ginger
- teaspoon orange zest
- 1 tablespoon rice vinegar
- 1 tablespoon cornstarch
- 2 green onions, thinly sliced
- Sesame seeds for garnish (optional

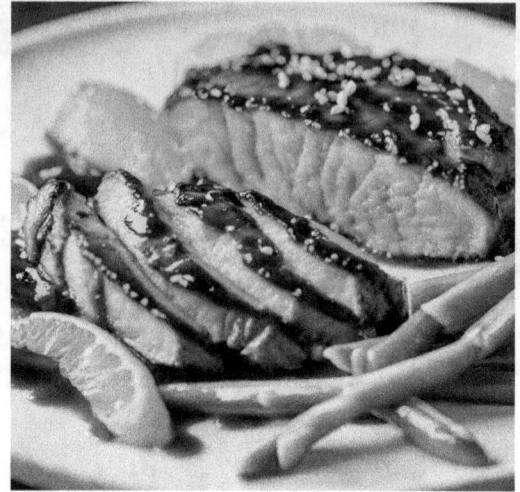

Instructions:
1. Preheat the oven to 400°F (200°C).
2. Score the skin of the duck breasts with a sharp knife in a crosshatch pattern, being careful not to cut into the meat.
3. Season the duck breasts generously with salt and pepper on both sides.
4. In a small saucepan, combine orange juice, soy sauce, honey, minced garlic, grated ginger, orange zest, and rice vinegar. Bring to a simmer over medium heat.
5. In a small bowl, mix cornstarch with 1 tablespoon of water to make a slurry.
6. Stir the cornstarch slurry into the simmering sauce and cook until thickened, about 2-3 minutes.
7. Place the duck breasts skin side down in a cold, oven-safe skillet.
8. Place the skillet over medium heat and cook for 6-8 minutes, or until the skin is golden brown and crispy. Flip the duck breasts and cook for an additional 2 minutes.
9. Transfer the skillet to the preheated oven and roast for 8-10 minutes, or until the duck breasts reach an internal temperature of 135°F (57°C) for medium-rare or desired doneness.
10. Remove the duck breasts from the oven and let them rest for a few minutes.
11. Slice the duck breasts thinly and drizzle with the orange glaze.
12. Garnish with sliced green onions and sesame seeds if desired.

- 13 Serve the Asian orange glazed duck breast hot with rice or vegetables.

Nutritional Information:
- Serving Size: 1 duck breast
- Servings: 4
- Calories per serving: approximately 350
- Total Fat: 20g
- Carbohydrates: 15g
- Fiber: 1g
- Protein: 25g

Cooking Time:
- Prep Time: 10 minutes
- Cooking Time: 20 minutes

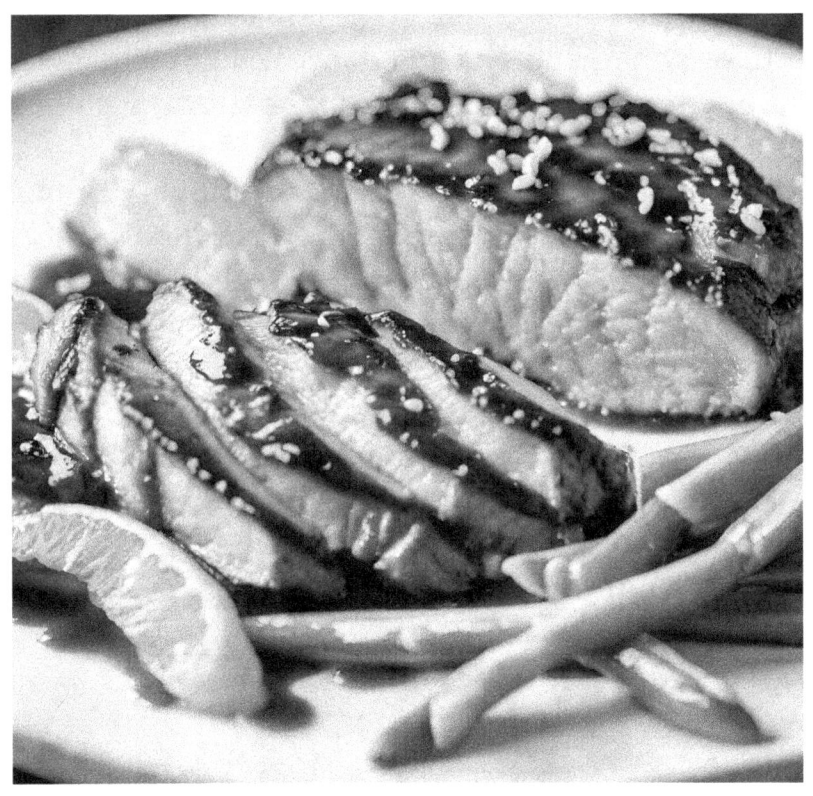

10. Italian Sausage and Kale Soup

Ingredients:
- 1 lb Italian sausage, casings removed
- 1 onion, chopped
- 2 cloves garlic, minced
- 4 cups chicken broth
- 1 can (14 oz) diced tomatoes
- 1 bunch kale, stems removed and leaves chopped
- 1 can (15 oz) cannellini beans, drained and rinsed
- 1 teaspoon dried oregano
- 1 teaspoon dried thyme
- Salt and pepper to taste
- Grated Parmesan cheese for garnish (optional)

Instructions:
1. In a large pot or Dutch oven, cook Italian sausage over medium heat until browned and crumbled, breaking it up with a spoon.
2. Add chopped onion to the pot and cook until softened, about 5 minutes.
3. Stir in minced garlic and cook for an additional 1 minute.
4. Add chicken broth, diced tomatoes (with juices), chopped kale, cannellini beans, dried oregano, and dried thyme to the pot.
5. Bring the soup to a simmer and cook for 15-20 minutes, or until the kale is tender and the flavors have melded.
6. Season with salt and pepper to taste.
7. Ladle the Italian sausage and kale soup into bowls.
8. Garnish with grated Parmesan cheese if desired.
9. Serve hot with crusty bread for dipping.

Nutritional Information:
- Serving Size: 1 cup
- Servings: 6
- Calories per serving: approximately 300
- Total Fat: 15g
- Carbohydrates: 20g
- Fiber: 5g
- Protein: 20g

Cooking Time:
- Prep Time: 10 minutes
- Cooking Time: 30 minutes

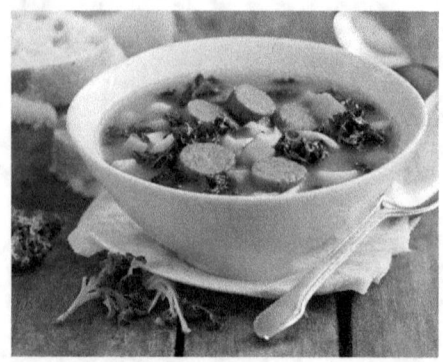

11. Thai Green Curry Beef

Ingredients:

- 1 lb beef sirloin, thinly sliced
- 1 can (14 oz) coconut milk
- 2 tablespoons Thai green curry paste
- 1 tablespoon fish sauce
- 1 tablespoon brown sugar
- 1 bell pepper, sliced
- 1 zucchini, sliced
- 1 carrot, sliced
- 1 cup green beans, trimmed
- Fresh basil leaves for garnish (optional)
- Cooked rice for serving

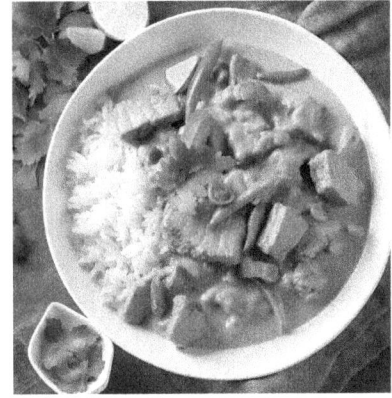

Instructions:

1. In a large skillet or wok, heat a small amount of coconut milk over medium heat.
2. Add Thai green curry paste to the skillet and stir-fry for 1-2 minutes until fragrant.
3. Stir in beef sirloin slices and cook until browned on all sides.
4. Pour in the remaining coconut milk, fish sauce, and brown sugar. Stir to combine.
5. Add sliced bell pepper, zucchini, carrot, and green beans to the skillet. Stir-fry for 5-7 minutes until the vegetables are tender-crisp.
6. Taste and adjust seasoning if necessary.
7. Remove from heat and garnish with fresh basil leaves if desired.
8. Serve the Thai green curry beef hot over cooked rice.

Nutritional Information:

- Serving Size: 1 cup curry with rice
- Servings: 4
- Calories per serving: approximately 350
- Total Fat: 20g
- Carbohydrates: 15g
- Fiber: 3g
- Protein: 25g

Cooking Time:

- Prep Time: 15 minutes
- Cooking Time: 20 minutes

12. Spanish Chicken and Chorizo Paella

Ingredients:
- 1 lb chicken thighs, bone-in and skin-on
- 6 oz chorizo sausage, sliced
- 1 onion, diced
- 2 cloves garlic, minced
- 1 bell pepper, diced
- 1 tomato, diced
- 1 1/2 cups Arborio rice
- 4 cups chicken broth
- 1 teaspoon smoked paprika
- 1 teaspoon saffron threads
- Salt and pepper to taste
- Fresh parsley for garnish (optional)
- Lemon wedges for serving

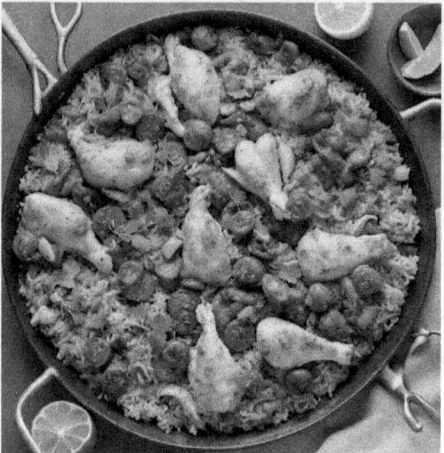

Instructions:
1. Season chicken thighs with salt, pepper, and smoked paprika.
2. In a large skillet or paella pan, heat olive oil over medium-high heat.
3. Add chicken thighs to the skillet and cook until browned on all sides. Remove from the skillet and set aside.
4. In the same skillet, add sliced chorizo sausage and cook until browned. Remove from the skillet and set aside.
5. Add diced onion, minced garlic, diced bell pepper, and diced tomato to the skillet. Cook until softened, about 5 minutes.
6. Stir in Arborio rice, smoked paprika, and saffron threads. Cook for 1-2 minutes until the rice is coated with the spices.
7. Pour chicken broth into the skillet and stir to combine. Arrange the browned chicken thighs and chorizo slices on top of the rice mixture.
8. Bring the mixture to a simmer, then reduce the heat to low. Cover and cook for 20-25 minutes, or until the rice is tender and the liquid is absorbed.
9. Remove from heat and let it rest, covered, for 5 minutes.
10. Garnish with fresh parsley if desired and serve with lemon wedges for squeezing over the paella.

Nutritional Information:
- Serving Size: 1/4 of the paella
- Servings: 4
- Calories per serving: approximately 450
- Total Fat: 20g
- Carbohydrates: 40g
- Fiber: 2g
- Protein: 25g

Cooking Time:
- Prep Time: 15 minutes
- Cooking Time: 35-40 minutes

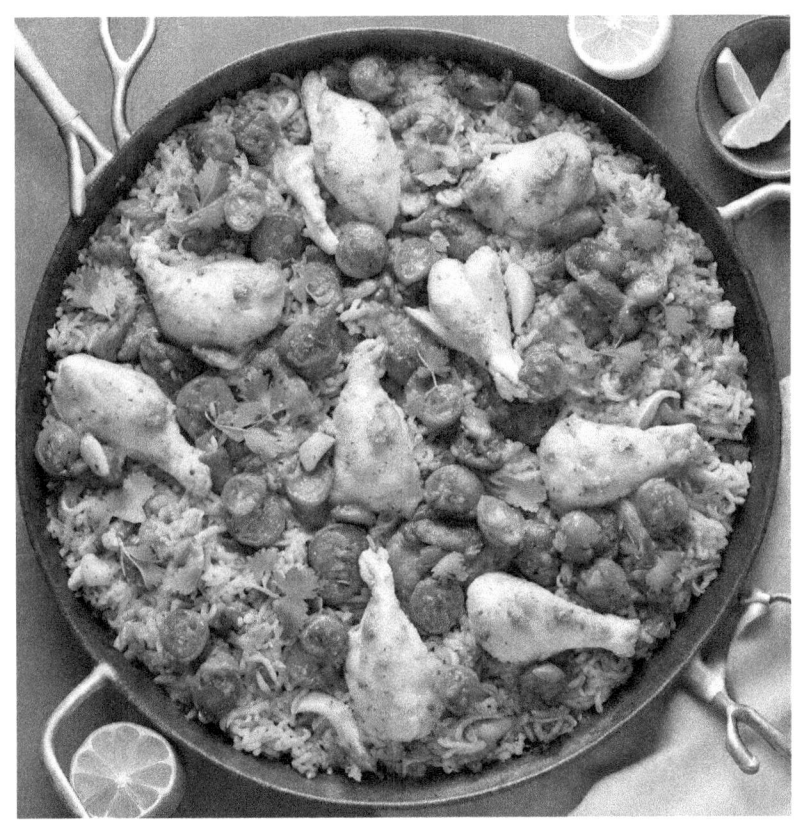

13. Barbecue Pulled Pork

Ingredients:

- 3 lbs pork shoulder (also known as pork butt), trimmed of excess fat
- 1 onion, sliced
- 4 cloves garlic, minced
- 1 cup barbecue sauce
- 1/4 cup apple cider vinegar
- 1/4 cup brown sugar
- 1 tablespoon Worcestershire sauce
- 1 tablespoon Dijon mustard
- 1 teaspoon smoked paprika
- 1/2 teaspoon cayenne pepper (optional)
- Salt and pepper to taste
- Hamburger buns or sandwich rolls for serving

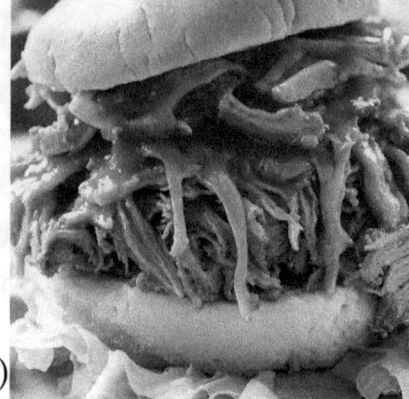

Instructions:
1. In a slow cooker, layer sliced onions on the bottom.
2. Place the pork shoulder on top of the onions.
3. In a bowl, mix together minced garlic, barbecue sauce, apple cider vinegar, brown sugar, Worcestershire sauce, Dijon mustard, smoked paprika, cayenne pepper (if using), salt, and pepper.
4. Pour the barbecue sauce mixture over the pork shoulder, ensuring it is well coated.
5. Cover and cook on low heat for 8-10 hours, or until the pork is tender and easily shreds with a fork.
6. Remove the pork shoulder from the slow cooker and shred it using two forks.
7. Return the shredded pork to the slow cooker and stir to coat with the barbecue sauce.
8. Serve the barbecue pulled pork on hamburger buns or sandwich rolls.

Nutritional Information:
- Serving Size: 1/2 cup pulled pork (without bun)
- Servings: 10
- Calories per serving: approximately 300

Total Fat: 15g Carbohydrates: 15g Fiber: 1g Protein: 25g

Cooking Time:
- Prep Time: 15 minutes Cooking Time: 8-10 hours (slow cooker)

14. Indian Butter Chicken (Murgh Makhani)

Ingredients:
- 1.5 lbs boneless, skinless chicken thighs, cut into bite-sized pieces
- 1 onion, finely chopped
- 4 cloves garlic, minced
- 1 tablespoon grated ginger
- 1 cup tomato puree
- 1/2 cup plain yogurt
- 1/4 cup heavy cream
- 2 tablespoons butter
- 1 tablespoon vegetable oil
- 1 tablespoon garam masala
- 1 teaspoon ground turmeric
- 1 teaspoon ground cumin
- 1 teaspoon ground coriander
- 1/2 teaspoon chili powder (adjust to taste)
- Salt to taste
- Chopped fresh cilantro for garnish (optional)
- Cooked rice or naan for serving

Instructions:
1. Heat vegetable oil in a large skillet or pan over medium heat.
2. Add chopped onion, minced garlic, and grated ginger to the skillet. Cook until onions are soft and translucent, about 5-7 minutes.
3. Stir in garam masala, ground turmeric, ground cumin, ground coriander, and chili powder. Cook for 1-2 minutes until fragrant.
4. Add tomato puree to the skillet and cook for another 5 minutes, stirring occasionally.
5. Stir in plain yogurt and heavy cream. Cook for an additional 2-3 minutes.
6. In a separate skillet, heat butter over medium-high heat. Add chicken pieces and cook until browned on all sides, about 5-7 minutes.
7. Transfer the browned chicken pieces to the tomato sauce mixture. Simmer for 10-15 minutes, stirring occasionally, until the chicken is cooked through and the sauce has thickened.
8. Season with salt to taste.
9. Garnish with chopped fresh cilantro if desired.
10. Serve the Indian butter chicken hot with rice or naan.

Nutritional Information:
- Serving Size: 1/4 of the recipe
- Servings: 4
- Calories per serving: approximately 400
- Total Fat: 25g
- Carbohydrates: 10g
- Fiber: 2g
- Protein: 30g

Cooking Time:
- Prep Time: 15 minutes
- Cooking Time: 30 minutes

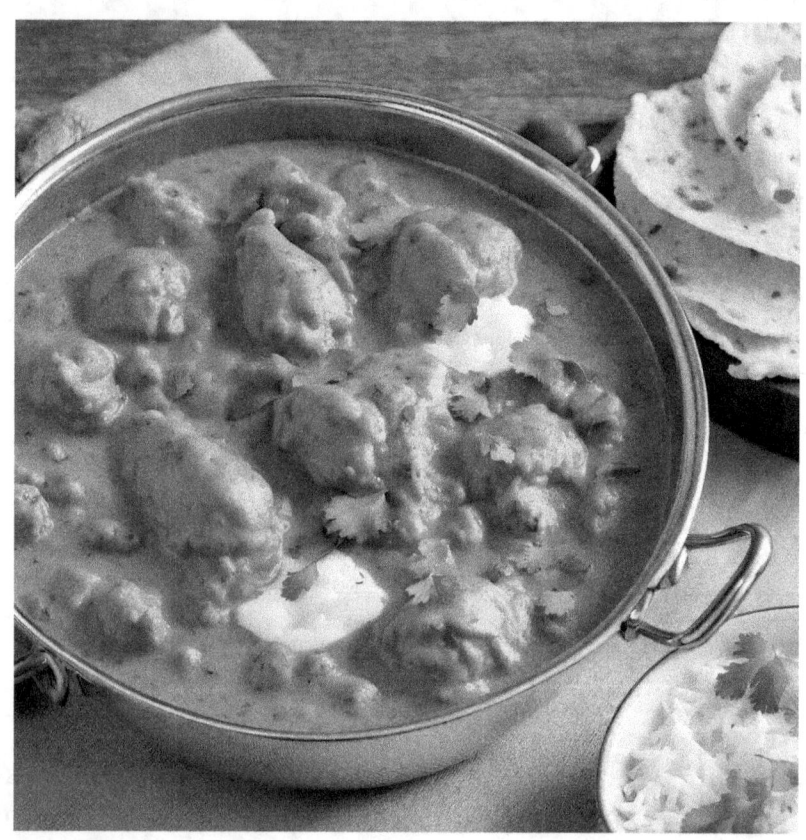

15. French Coq au Vin

Ingredients:
- 4 chicken legs (thighs and drumsticks), skin-on
- 4 slices bacon, chopped
- 1 onion, chopped
- 2 carrots, chopped
- 2 cloves garlic, minced
- 8 oz mushrooms, sliced
- 1 cup red wine (such as Burgundy or Pinot Noir)
- 1 cup chicken broth
- 2 tablespoons tomato paste
- 2 tablespoons all-purpose flour
- 2 tablespoons butter
- 1 tablespoon olive oil
- 2 sprigs fresh thyme
- 2 bay leaves
- Salt and pepper to taste
- Chopped fresh parsley for garnish (optional)
- Mashed potatoes or crusty bread for serving

Instructions:
1. Season chicken legs with salt and pepper.
2. In a large Dutch oven or heavy-bottomed pot, heat olive oil over medium-high heat.
3. Add chicken legs to the pot and cook until browned on all sides, about 8-10 minutes. Remove from the pot and set aside.
4. In the same pot, add chopped bacon and cook until crispy.
5. Add chopped onion, carrots, and minced garlic to the pot. Cook until vegetables are softened, about 5 minutes.
6. Stir in sliced mushrooms and cook for an additional 3-4 minutes.
7. Sprinkle flour over the vegetables and cook, stirring constantly, for 2 minutes.
8. Slowly pour in red wine and chicken broth, stirring to combine and scraping up any browned bits from the bottom of the pot.
9. Stir in tomato paste until well incorporated.
10. Return the chicken legs to the pot along with fresh thyme sprigs and bay leaves.

- 12 Bring the mixture to a simmer, then reduce the heat to low. Cover and cook for 1 to 1 1/2 hours, or until the chicken is cooked through and tender.
- Once the chicken is cooked, remove it from the pot and set aside.
- Simmer the sauce uncovered for an additional 10-15 minutes, or until slightly thickened.
- Stir in butter until melted and incorporated into the sauce.
- Return the chicken to the pot and simmer for a few more minutes to heat through.
- Remove the bay leaves and thyme sprigs.
- Garnish with chopped fresh parsley if desired.
- Serve the French Coq au Vin hot with mashed potatoes or crusty bread.

Nutritional Information:
- Serving Size: 1 chicken leg with sauce
- Servings: 4
- Calories per serving: approximately 400
- Total Fat: 20g
- Carbohydrates: 10g
- Fiber: 2g
- Protein: 35g

Cooking Time:
- Prep Time: 20 minutes
- Cooking Time: 2 to 2 1/2 hours

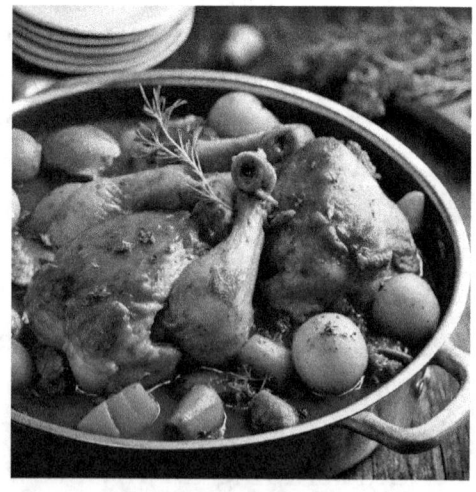

16. Chipotle Lime Grilled Shrimp

Ingredients:
- 1 lb large shrimp, peeled and deveined
- 2 tablespoons olive oil
- 2 chipotle peppers in adobo sauce, minced
- Zest and juice of 1 lime
- 2 cloves garlic, minced
- 1 teaspoon ground cumin
- 1/2 teaspoon chili powder
- Salt and pepper to taste
- Chopped fresh cilantro for garnish (optional)
- Lime wedges for serving

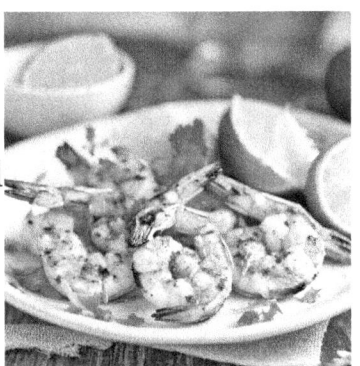

Instructions:
1. In a bowl, whisk together olive oil, minced chipotle peppers, lime zest, lime juice, minced garlic, ground cumin, chili powder, salt, and pepper to make the marinade.
2. Add peeled and deveined shrimp to the marinade and toss to coat evenly. Let marinate in the refrigerator for 20-30 minutes.
3. Preheat grill to medium-high heat.
4. Thread marinated shrimp onto skewers.
5. Grill the shrimp skewers for 2-3 minutes per side, or until opaque and slightly charred.
6. Remove from the grill and let them rest for a few minutes.
7. Garnish with chopped fresh cilantro if desired.
8. Serve the chipotle lime grilled shrimp hot with lime wedges.

Nutritional Information:
- Serving Size: 1/4 lb shrimp
- Servings: 4
- Calories per serving: approximately 150
- Total Fat: 7g
- Carbohydrates: 2g
- Fiber: 0g
- Protein: 20g

Cooking Time:
- Prep Time: 10 minutes (plus marinating time)
- Cooking Time: 5-6 minutes

17. Sesame Ginger Turkey Stir-Fry

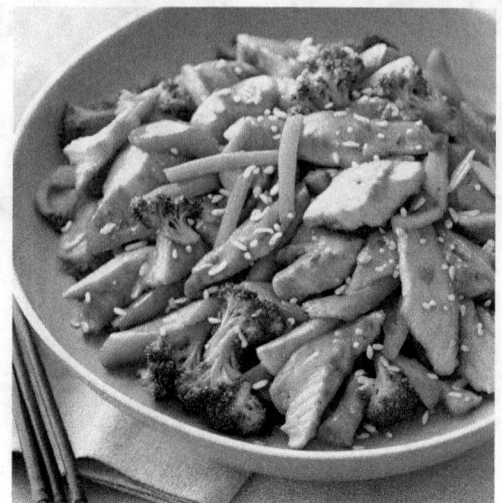

Ingredients:
- 1 lb turkey breast, thinly sliced
- 2 tablespoons soy sauce
- 1 tablespoon sesame oil
- 1 tablespoon rice vinegar
- 1 tablespoon honey
- 2 cloves garlic, minced
- 1 tablespoon fresh ginger, grated
- 1 tablespoon cornstarch
- 2 tablespoons vegetable oil
- 1 bell pepper, sliced
- 1 cup snow peas
- 1 carrot, julienned
- Cooked rice for serving
- Sesame seeds for garnish (optional)
- Chopped green onions for garnish (optional)

Instructions:
1. In a bowl, whisk together soy sauce, sesame oil, rice vinegar, honey, minced garlic, grated ginger, and cornstarch to make the marinade.
2. Add thinly sliced turkey breast to the marinade and toss to coat evenly. Let marinate in the refrigerator for 20-30 minutes.
3. Heat vegetable oil in a large skillet or wok over high heat.
4. Add marinated turkey slices to the skillet and stir-fry for 2-3 minutes until browned and cooked through. Remove from the skillet and set aside.
5. In the same skillet, add sliced bell pepper, snow peas, and julienned carrot. Stir-fry for 3-4 minutes until vegetables are tender-crisp.
6. Return the cooked turkey to the skillet and toss with the vegetables to combine.
7. Serve the sesame ginger turkey stir-fry hot over cooked rice.
8. Garnish with sesame seeds and chopped green onions if desired.

Nutritional Information:
- Serving Size: 1/4 of the stir-fry
- Servings: 4
- Calories per serving: approximately 250
- Total Fat: 10g Carbohydrates: 15g Fiber: 3g Protein: 25g

Cooking Time: 30 minutes

18. Greek Lemon Garlic Lamb Chops

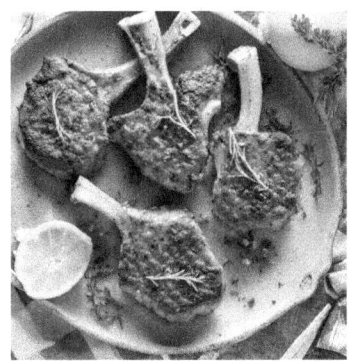

Ingredients:
- 8 lamb loin chops
- 1/4 cup olive oil
- Zest and juice of 1 lemon
- 4 cloves garlic, minced
- 1 tablespoon dried oregano
- Salt and pepper to taste
- Chopped fresh parsley for garnish (optional)

Instructions:
1. In a bowl, whisk together olive oil, lemon zest, lemon juice, minced garlic, dried oregano, salt, and pepper to make the marinade.
2. Add lamb loin chops to the marinade and toss to coat evenly. Let marinate in the refrigerator for 30 minutes to 1 hour.
3. Preheat grill or grill pan to medium-high heat.
4. Remove lamb chops from the marinade and shake off any excess.
5. Grill the lamb chops for 3-4 minutes per side for medium-rare, or until cooked to your desired doneness.
6. Remove from the grill and let them rest for a few minutes.
7. Garnish with chopped fresh parsley if desired.
8. Serve the Greek lemon garlic lamb chops hot.

Nutritional Information:
- Serving Size: 2 lamb chops
- Servings: 4
- Calories per serving: approximately 400
- Total Fat: 30g
- Carbohydrates: 2g
- Fiber: 0g
- Protein: 30g

Cooking Time:
- Prep Time: 10 minutes (plus marinating time)
- Cooking Time: 8-10 minutes

19. Honey Mustard Glazed Salmon

Ingredients:
- 4 salmon fillets
- 1/4 cup Dijon mustard
- 2 tablespoons honey
- 1 tablespoon olive oil
- 1 tablespoon lemon juice
- 2 cloves garlic, minced
- Salt and pepper to taste
- Chopped fresh parsley for garnish (optional)
- Lemon wedges for serving

Instructions:
1. Preheat oven to 400°F (200°C).
2. In a bowl, whisk together Dijon mustard, honey, olive oil, lemon juice, minced garlic, salt, and pepper to make the glaze.
3. Place salmon fillets on a baking sheet lined with parchment paper.
4. Brush the salmon fillets generously with the honey mustard glaze.
5. Bake in the preheated oven for 12-15 minutes, or until the salmon is cooked through and flakes easily with a fork.
6. Remove from the oven and let them rest for a few minutes.
7. Garnish with chopped fresh parsley if desired.
8. Serve the honey mustard glazed salmon hot with lemon wedges.

Nutritional Information:
- Serving Size: 1 salmon fillet
- Servings: 4
- Calories per serving: approximately 300
- Total Fat: 15g
- Carbohydrates: 10g
- Fiber: 0g
- Protein: 25g

Cooking Time:
- Prep Time: 5 minutes
- Cooking Time: 20 minutes

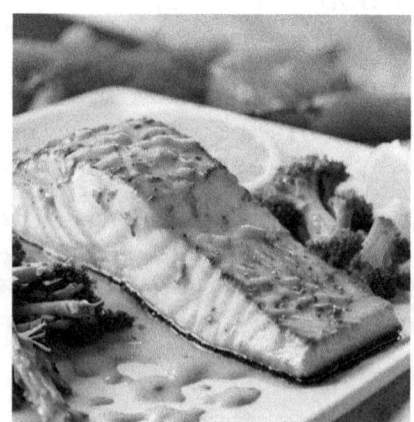

20. Italian Meatballs

Ingredients:
- 1 lb ground beef
- 1/2 cup breadcrumbs
- 1/4 cup grated Parmesan cheese
- 1/4 cup chopped fresh parsley
- 1 egg
- 2 cloves garlic, minced
- 1 teaspoon dried oregano
- 1 teaspoon dried basil
- Salt and pepper to taste
- Olive oil for cooking
- Marinara sauce for serving

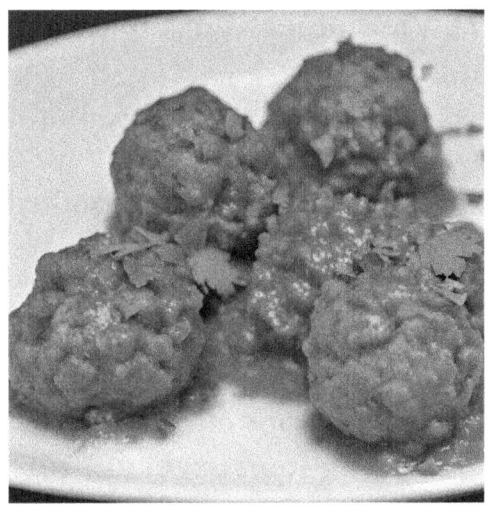

Instructions:
1. Preheat oven to 400°F (200°C).
2. In a large mixing bowl, combine ground beef, breadcrumbs, Parmesan cheese, chopped parsley, egg, minced garlic, dried oregano, dried basil, salt, and pepper. Mix until well combined.
3. Shape the mixture into meatballs of desired size.
4. Heat olive oil in a large skillet over medium heat.
5. Add the meatballs to the skillet and cook until browned on all sides, about 2-3 minutes per side.
6. Transfer the browned meatballs to a baking sheet lined with parchment paper.
7. Bake in the preheated oven for 10-12 minutes, or until the meatballs are cooked through.
8. Serve the Italian meatballs hot with marinara sauce.

Nutritional Information:
- Serving Size: 4 meatballs
- Servings: 4
- Calories per serving: approximately 300
- Total Fat: 20g
- Carbohydrates: 10g
- Fiber: 1g
- Protein: 20g

Cooking Time:
- Prep Time: 15 minutes
- Cooking Time: 15 minutes

21. Vietnamese Lemongrass Chicken

Ingredients:
- 1 lb chicken thighs, boneless and skinless, cut into bite-sized pieces
- 2 stalks lemongrass, outer layers removed, finely chopped
- 3 cloves garlic, minced
- 2 shallots, finely chopped
- 1 tablespoon fish sauce
- 1 tablespoon soy sauce
- 1 tablespoon honey
- 1 tablespoon vegetable oil
- 1 teaspoon sesame oil
- 1/2 teaspoon ground black pepper
- Fresh cilantro for garnish (optional)
- Cooked rice for serving

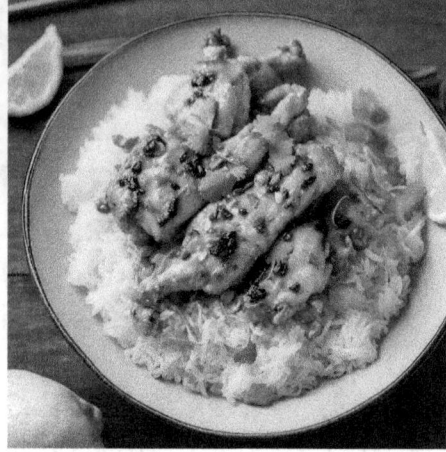

Instructions:
1. In a bowl, combine chopped lemongrass, minced garlic, chopped shallots, fish sauce, soy sauce, honey, vegetable oil, sesame oil, and black pepper to make the marinade.
2. Add chicken thigh pieces to the marinade and toss to coat evenly. Let marinate in the refrigerator for at least 30 minutes.
3. Heat a skillet or grill pan over medium-high heat.
4. Add marinated chicken thigh pieces to the skillet and cook for 6-8 minutes, turning occasionally, until browned and cooked through.
5. Remove from heat and let them rest for a few minutes.
6. Garnish with fresh cilantro if desired.
7. Serve the Vietnamese lemongrass chicken hot with cooked rice.

Nutritional Information:
- Serving Size: 1/4 of the chicken
- Servings: 4
- Calories per serving: approximately 250
- Total Fat: 10g
- Carbohydrates: 10g
- Fiber: 1g
- Protein: 25g

Cooking Time:
- Prep Time: 10 minutes (plus marinating time)
- Cooking Time: 10 minutes

22. Herb-Roasted Cornish Hens

Ingredients:
- 2 Cornish hens
- 2 tablespoons olive oil
- 2 cloves garlic, minced
- 1 tablespoon chopped fresh rosemary
- 1 tablespoon chopped fresh thyme
- 1 tablespoon chopped fresh parsley
- Salt and pepper to taste
- Lemon wedges for serving

Instructions:
1. Preheat oven to 375°F (190°C).
2. In a small bowl, mix together olive oil, minced garlic, chopped rosemary, chopped thyme, chopped parsley, salt, and pepper to make the herb mixture.
3. Pat the Cornish hens dry with paper towels.
4. Rub the herb mixture all over the Cornish hens, ensuring they are thoroughly coated.
5. Place the Cornish hens in a roasting pan or baking dish.
6. Roast in the preheated oven for 50-60 minutes, or until the internal temperature reaches 165°F (74°C) when measured with a meat thermometer.
7. Remove from the oven and let them rest for 5-10 minutes before serving.
8. Serve the herb-roasted Cornish hens hot with lemon wedges.

Nutritional Information:
- Serving Size: 1/2 Cornish hen
- Servings: 4
- Calories per serving: approximately 400
- Total Fat: 25g
- Carbohydrates: 0g
- Fiber: 0g
- Protein: 40g

Cooking Time:
- Prep Time: 10 minutes
- Cooking Time: 50-60 minutes

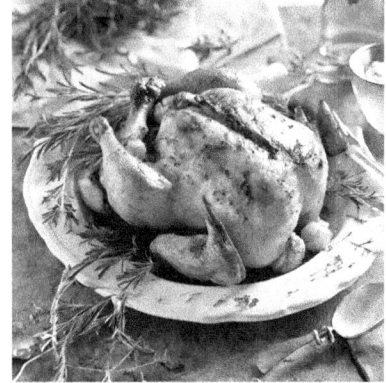

23. Thai Basil Chicken

Ingredients:
- 1 lb chicken breast or thighs, thinly sliced
- 2 tablespoons vegetable oil
- 3 cloves garlic, minced
- 2 shallots, thinly sliced
- 2 red chilies, thinly sliced
- 1 bell pepper, thinly sliced
- 1 cup fresh basil leaves
- 2 tablespoons oyster sauce
- 1 tablespoon soy sauce
- 1 tablespoon fish sauce
- 1 teaspoon sugar
- Cooked rice for serving

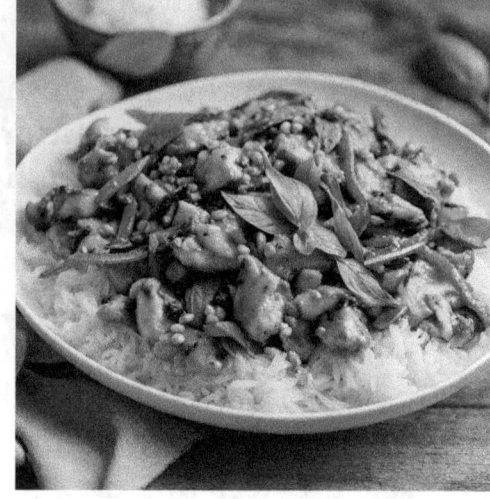

Instructions:
1. Heat vegetable oil in a wok or large skillet over medium-high heat.
2. Add minced garlic, thinly sliced shallots, and sliced red chilies to the wok. Stir-fry for 1-2 minutes until fragrant.
3. Add thinly sliced chicken to the wok and stir-fry for 3-4 minutes until browned and cooked through.
4. Stir in thinly sliced bell pepper and continue to stir-fry for another 2 minutes.
5. Add oyster sauce, soy sauce, fish sauce, and sugar to the wok. Stir to combine.
6. Remove the wok from heat and stir in fresh basil leaves until wilted.
7. Serve the Thai basil chicken hot over cooked rice.

Nutritional Information:
- Serving Size: 1/4 of the chicken
- Servings: 4
- Calories per serving: approximately 250
- Total Fat: 10g
- Carbohydrates: 10g
- Fiber: 1g
- Protein: 25g

Cooking Time:
- Prep Time: 10 minutes
- Cooking Time: 10 minutes

FISH AND SEAFOOD RECIPES

1. Japanese Chirashi Sushi
Ingredients:
- 2 cups sushi rice
- 2 1/2 cups water
- 1/4 cup rice vinegar
- 2 tablespoons sugar
- 1 teaspoon salt
- Assorted sashimi (such as tuna, salmon, yellowtail), thinly sliced
- Assorted vegetables (such as cucumber, avocado, radish), thinly sliced
- Nori seaweed strips
- Soy sauce, for serving
- Wasabi, for serving
- Pickled ginger, for serving

Instructions:
1. Rinse the sushi rice under cold water until the water runs clear. Drain well.
2. In a rice cooker or pot, combine the sushi rice and water. Cook according to the rice cooker instructions or bring to a boil, then reduce heat to low, cover, and simmer for 18-20 minutes until the rice is cooked and water is absorbed.
3. In a small saucepan, combine rice vinegar, sugar, and salt. Heat over low heat until the sugar and salt dissolve. Remove from heat and let it cool.
4. Transfer the cooked rice to a large bowl and gently fold in the seasoned vinegar mixture. Allow the rice to cool to room temperature.
5. Arrange the sliced sashimi, vegetables, and nori strips on top of the sushi rice in a decorative pattern.
6. Serve the Japanese chirashi sushi with soy sauce, wasabi, and pickled ginger on the side.

Nutritional Information:
- Serving Size: 1/4 of the recipe
- Servings: 4
- Calories per serving: approximately 400
- Total Fat: 5g Carbohydrates: 75g Fiber: 2g Protein: 15g

Cooking Time: 50 Minutes

2. Italian Cioppino

Ingredients:
- 1 lb mixed seafood (such as shrimp, mussels, clams, squid), cleaned and deveined
- 2 tablespoons olive oil
- 1 onion, chopped
- 3 cloves garlic, minced
- 1/2 cup white wine
- 1 can (28 oz) crushed tomatoes
- 2 cups seafood broth or fish stock
- 1/4 cup chopped fresh parsley
- 1 teaspoon dried oregano
- Salt and pepper to taste
- Crushed red pepper flakes (optional)
- Sliced crusty bread for serving

Instructions:
1. Heat olive oil in a large pot or Dutch oven over medium heat.
2. Add chopped onion and minced garlic to the pot. Cook until softened, about 3-4 minutes.
3. Pour in white wine and cook for 2 minutes, allowing the alcohol to evaporate.
4. Stir in crushed tomatoes, seafood broth, chopped parsley, dried oregano, salt, pepper, and crushed red pepper flakes (if using).
5. Bring the mixture to a simmer and let it cook for 15-20 minutes to allow the flavors to meld together.
6. Add the mixed seafood to the pot and cook for an additional 5-7 minutes until the seafood is cooked through.
7. Taste and adjust seasoning if needed.
8. Serve the Italian cioppino hot with sliced crusty bread.

Nutritional Information:
- Serving Size: 1/4 of the recipe
- Servings: 4
- Calories per serving: approximately 250
- Total Fat: 8g
- Carbohydrates: 20g
- Fiber: 4g
- Protein: 20g

Cooking Time: 45 minutes

3. Thai Green Curry Mussels

Ingredients:
- 2 lbs fresh mussels, cleaned and debearded
- 2 tablespoons green curry paste
- 1 can (13.5 oz) coconut milk
- 1 cup seafood broth or fish stock
- 1 red bell pepper, thinly sliced
- 1 onion, thinly sliced
- 2 tablespoons fish sauce
- 1 tablespoon brown sugar
- Juice of 1 lime
- Fresh cilantro for garnish (optional)
- Cooked rice or crusty bread for serving

Instructions:
1. In a large pot or Dutch oven, heat green curry paste over medium heat for 1-2 minutes until fragrant.
2. Pour in coconut milk and seafood broth. Stir to combine.
3. Add thinly sliced red bell pepper and onion to the pot. Cook for 3-4 minutes until slightly softened.
4. Stir in fish sauce and brown sugar.
5. Add cleaned mussels to the pot and cover with a lid. Cook for 5-7 minutes until the mussels have opened.
6. Discard any mussels that have not opened.
7. Squeeze lime juice over the mussels and stir gently to combine.
8. Garnish with fresh cilantro if desired.
9. Serve the Thai green curry mussels hot with cooked rice or crusty bread.

Nutritional Information:
- Serving Size: 1/4 of the recipe
- Servings: 4
- Calories per serving: approximately 300
- Total Fat: 12g
- Carbohydrates: 20g
- Fiber: 2g
- Protein: 20g

Cooking Time:
- Prep Time: 10 minutes
- Cooking Time: 15 minutes

4. American Grilled Halibut with Lemon and Herbs

Ingredients:
- 4 halibut fillets
- 2 tablespoons olive oil
- Zest and juice of 1 lemon
- 2 cloves garlic, minced
- 1 tablespoon chopped fresh parsley
- 1 tablespoon chopped fresh dill
- Salt and pepper to taste
- Lemon wedges for serving

Instructions:
1. Preheat grill to medium-high heat.
2. In a bowl, whisk together olive oil, lemon zest, lemon juice, minced garlic, chopped parsley, chopped dill, salt, and pepper to make the marinade.
3. Pat the halibut fillets dry with paper towels and place them in a shallow dish.
4. Pour the marinade over the halibut fillets, turning to coat evenly. Let marinate for 15-20 minutes.
5. Remove the halibut fillets from the marinade and shake off any excess.
6. Grill the halibut fillets for 3-4 minutes per side, or until the fish is opaque and flakes easily with a fork.
7. Remove from the grill and let them rest for a few minutes.
8. Serve the grilled halibut hot with lemon wedges.

Nutritional Information:
- Serving Size: 1 fillet
- Servings: 4
- Calories per serving: approximately 200
- Total Fat: 10g
- Carbohydrates: 1g
- Fiber: 0g
- Protein: 25g

Cooking Time:
- Prep Time: 10 minutes (plus marinating time)
- Cooking Time: 8-10 minutes

5. Greek Grilled Shrimp Souvlaki

Ingredients:
- 1 lb large shrimp, peeled and deveined
- 1/4 cup olive oil
- 3 cloves garlic, minced
- 1 tablespoon chopped fresh oregano
- 1 tablespoon chopped fresh parsley
- Zest and juice of 1 lemon
- Salt and pepper to taste
- Wooden skewers, soaked in water
- Tzatziki sauce for serving
- Pita bread for serving
- Sliced red onion, sliced cucumber, and tomato wedges for serving

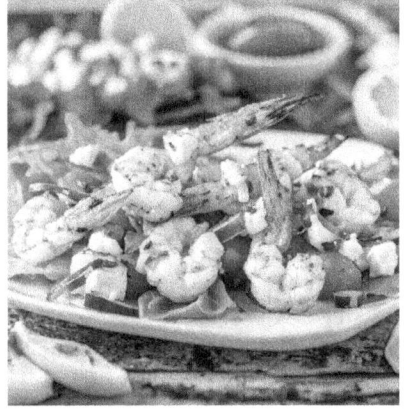

Instructions:
1. In a bowl, combine olive oil, minced garlic, chopped oregano, chopped parsley, lemon zest, lemon juice, salt, and pepper to make the marinade.
2. Add peeled and deveined shrimp to the marinade and toss to coat evenly. Let marinate in the refrigerator for 30 minutes to 1 hour.
3. Preheat grill to medium-high heat.
4. Thread marinated shrimp onto soaked wooden skewers.
5. Grill the shrimp skewers for 2-3 minutes per side, or until pink and cooked through.
6. Remove from the grill and let them rest for a few minutes.
7. Serve the Greek grilled shrimp souvlaki hot with tzatziki sauce, pita bread, sliced red onion, sliced cucumber, and tomato wedges.

Nutritional Information:
- Serving Size: 1/4 of the recipe
- Servings: 4
- Calories per serving: approximately 200
- Total Fat: 10g
- Carbohydrates: 3g
- Fiber: 1g Protein: 25g

Cooking Time:
- Prep Time: 10 minutes (plus marinating time)
- Cooking Time: 6-8 minutes

6. Japanese Sushi Nigiri

Ingredients:
- 1 cup sushi rice
- 2 cups water
- 2 tablespoons rice vinegar
- 1 tablespoon sugar
- 1/2 teaspoon salt
- Assorted sushi-grade fish (such as tuna, salmon, yellowtail), thinly sliced
- Wasabi paste
- Soy sauce for dipping
- Pickled ginger for serving

Instructions:
1. Rinse the sushi rice under cold water until the water runs clear. Drain well.
2. In a rice cooker or pot, combine the sushi rice and water. Cook according to the rice cooker instructions or bring to a boil, then reduce heat to low, cover, and simmer for 18-20 minutes until the rice is cooked and water is absorbed.
3. In a small saucepan, combine rice vinegar, sugar, and salt. Heat over low heat until the sugar and salt dissolve. Remove from heat and let it cool.
4. Transfer the cooked rice to a large bowl and gently fold in the seasoned vinegar mixture. Allow the rice to cool to room temperature.
5. With wet hands, shape the sushi rice into small oblong shapes.
6. Place a slice of sushi-grade fish on top of each rice mound.
7. Serve the Japanese sushi nigiri with wasabi paste, soy sauce for dipping, and pickled ginger.

Nutritional Information:
- Serving Size: 2 pieces of nigiri
- Servings: 4
- Calories per serving: approximately 200
- Total Fat: 2g
- Carbohydrates: 40g
- Fiber: 1g   Protein: 8g

Cooking Time:
- Prep Time: 15 minutes
- Cooking Time: 20 minutes

7. Italian Baked Cod with Cherry Tomatoes and Olives

Ingredients:
- 4 cod fillets
- 2 cups cherry tomatoes, halved
- 1/2 cup pitted Kalamata olives
- 3 cloves garlic, thinly sliced
- 2 tablespoons olive oil
- 1 tablespoon balsamic vinegar
- 1 tablespoon chopped fresh basil
- Salt and pepper to taste
- Lemon wedges for serving

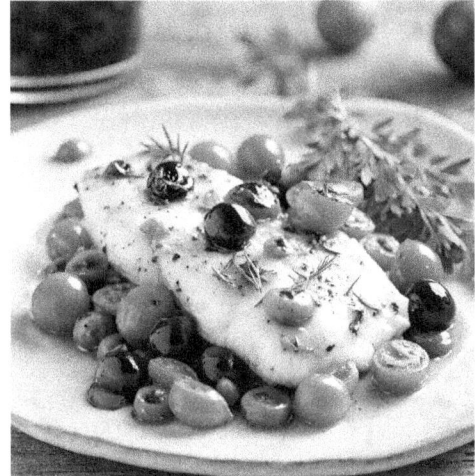

Instructions:
1. Preheat oven to 400°F (200°C).
2. Place cod fillets in a baking dish.
3. In a bowl, combine halved cherry tomatoes, pitted Kalamata olives, thinly sliced garlic, olive oil, balsamic vinegar, chopped basil, salt, and pepper. Toss to coat.
4. Spoon the tomato and olive mixture over the cod fillets.
5. Bake in the preheated oven for 15-20 minutes, or until the cod is cooked through and flakes easily with a fork.
6. Remove from the oven and let them rest for a few minutes.
7. Serve the Italian baked cod hot with lemon wedges.

Nutritional Information:
- Serving Size: 1 cod fillet with toppings
- Servings: 4
- Calories per serving: approximately 200
- Total Fat: 8g
- Carbohydrates: 10g
- Fiber: 2g
- Protein: 25g

Cooking Time:
- Prep Time: 10 minutes
- Cooking Time: 15-20 minutes

8. Thai Fish Cakes (Tod Mun Pla)

Ingredients:
- 1 lb white fish fillets, deboned and roughly chopped
- 1 tablespoon red curry paste
- 2 tablespoons fish sauce
- 1 tablespoon palm sugar or brown sugar
- 1 egg
- 1 tablespoon cornstarch
- 2 kaffir lime leaves, finely chopped
- 1/4 cup green beans, finely chopped
- Vegetable oil for frying
- Sweet chili sauce for serving
- Cucumber slices for serving

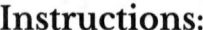

Instructions:
1. In a food processor, combine the white fish fillets, red curry paste, fish sauce, palm sugar, egg, and cornstarch. Process until well combined.
2. Transfer the mixture to a bowl and stir in chopped kaffir lime leaves and green beans.
3. Heat vegetable oil in a frying pan over medium heat.
4. Form the fish mixture into small patties and fry in the hot oil until golden brown and cooked through, about 3-4 minutes per side.
5. Remove the fish cakes from the oil and drain on paper towels.
6. Serve the Thai fish cakes hot with sweet chili sauce and cucumber slices.

Nutritional Information:
- Serving Size: 2 fish cakes
- Servings: 4
- Calories per serving: approximately 200
- Total Fat: 10g
- Carbohydrates: 10g
- Fiber: 1g
- Protein: 20g

Cooking Time:
- Prep Time: 15 minutes
- Cooking Time: 10 minutes

9. Spanish Garlic Butter Shrimp

Ingredients:
- 1 lb large shrimp, peeled and deveined
- 4 tablespoons unsalted butter
- 6 cloves garlic, minced
- 1 teaspoon smoked paprika
- 1/2 teaspoon red pepper flakes (optional)
- Salt and pepper to taste
- Chopped fresh parsley for garnish
- Lemon wedges for serving

Instructions:
1. Heat butter in a large skillet over medium heat.
2. Add minced garlic to the skillet and sauté until fragrant, about 1-2 minutes.
3. Add smoked paprika and red pepper flakes (if using) to the skillet and stir to combine.
4. Add peeled and deveined shrimp to the skillet and season with salt and pepper. Cook for 2-3 minutes per side, or until the shrimp is pink and cooked through.
5. Remove from heat and garnish with chopped fresh parsley.
6. Serve the Spanish garlic butter shrimp hot with lemon wedges.

Nutritional Information:
- Serving Size: 1/4 of the recipe
- Servings: 4
- Calories per serving: approximately 200
- Total Fat: 10g
- Carbohydrates: 2g
- Fiber: 0g
- Protein: 25g

Cooking Time:
- Prep Time: 10 minutes
- Cooking Time: 5-6 minutes

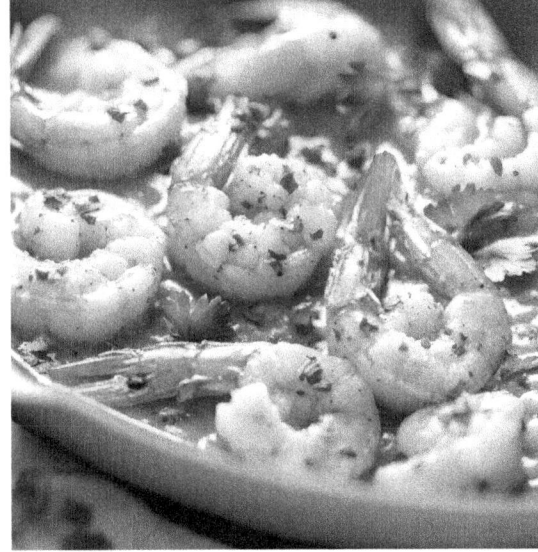

10. Japanese Grilled Miso Glazed Salmon

Ingredients:
- 4 salmon fillets
- 1/4 cup white miso paste
- 2 tablespoons soy sauce
- 2 tablespoons mirin
- 1 tablespoon sake (optional)
- 1 tablespoon honey
- 2 cloves garlic, minced
- 1 teaspoon grated ginger
- Sesame seeds for garnish
- Sliced green onions for garnish

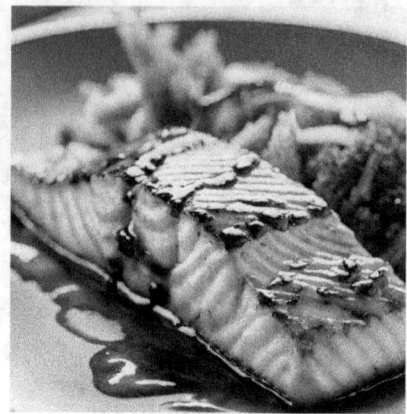

Instructions:
1. In a bowl, whisk together white miso paste, soy sauce, mirin, sake (if using), honey, minced garlic, and grated ginger to make the miso glaze.
2. Place salmon fillets in a shallow dish and pour the miso glaze over them. Marinate for at least 30 minutes, up to 2 hours.
3. Preheat grill to medium-high heat.
4. Remove salmon fillets from the marinade and shake off excess marinade.
5. Grill the salmon fillets for 4-5 minutes per side, or until the fish flakes easily with a fork and is cooked through.
6. Remove from the grill and let them rest for a few minutes.
7. Garnish with sesame seeds and sliced green onions.
8. Serve the Japanese grilled miso glazed salmon hot.

Nutritional Information:
- Serving Size: 1 salmon fillet
- Servings: 4
- Calories per serving: approximately 300
- Total Fat: 15g
- Carbohydrates: 10g
- Fiber: 1g
- Protein: 25g

Cooking Time:
- Prep Time: 10 minutes (plus marinating time)
- Cooking Time: 10 minutes

11. French Trout Almondine

Ingredients:
- 4 trout fillets
- 1/2 cup all-purpose flour
- Salt and pepper to taste
- 4 tablespoons unsalted butter
- 1/4 cup sliced almonds
- 2 tablespoons lemon juice
- 2 tablespoons chopped fresh parsley
- Lemon wedges for serving

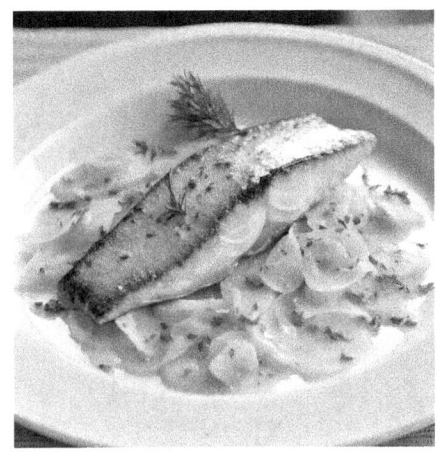

Instructions:
1. Season the all-purpose flour with salt and pepper on a plate.
2. Dredge the trout fillets in the seasoned flour, shaking off any excess.
3. In a large skillet, heat unsalted butter over medium heat.
4. Add trout fillets to the skillet and cook for 3-4 minutes per side, or until the fish is cooked through and golden brown.
5. Remove the trout fillets from the skillet and set aside.
6. In the same skillet, add sliced almonds and cook until golden brown and fragrant, about 1-2 minutes.
7. Stir in lemon juice and chopped fresh parsley.
8. Pour the almond and lemon mixture over the cooked trout fillets.
9. Serve the French trout almondine hot with lemon wedges.

Nutritional Information:
- Serving Size: 1 trout fillet
- Servings: 4
- Calories per serving: approximately 250
- Total Fat: 15g
- Carbohydrates: 6g
- Fiber: 1g
- Protein: 25g

Cooking Time:
- Prep Time: 10 minutes
- Cooking Time: 10 minutes

12. Thai Coconut Lime Shrimp Soup

Ingredients:
- 1 lb shrimp, peeled and deveined
- 2 cans (13.5 oz each) coconut milk
- 2 cups seafood broth or chicken broth
- 2 stalks lemongrass, bruised
- 3 kaffir lime leaves
- 2 inches galangal or ginger, sliced
- 2 red chilies, thinly sliced
- 2 tablespoons fish sauce
- 1 tablespoon brown sugar
- Juice of 2 limes
- 1 cup cherry tomatoes, halved
- Fresh cilantro for garnish
- Sliced green onions for garnish

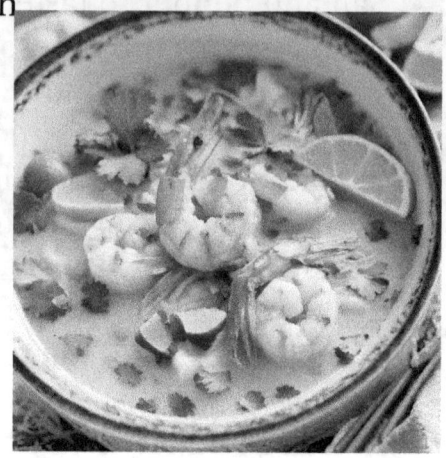

Instructions:
1. In a large pot, combine coconut milk and seafood broth.
2. Add bruised lemongrass, kaffir lime leaves, galangal or ginger slices, and thinly sliced red chilies to the pot.
3. Bring the mixture to a simmer over medium heat and let it cook for 10 minutes to infuse the flavors.
4. Stir in fish sauce, brown sugar, and lime juice.
5. Add peeled and deveined shrimp to the pot and cook for 3-4 minutes until the shrimp is pink and cooked through.
6. Stir in halved cherry tomatoes.
7. Remove lemongrass stalks, kaffir lime leaves, and galangal or ginger slices from the soup.
8. Ladle the Thai coconut lime shrimp soup into bowls and garnish with fresh cilantro and sliced green onions.
9. Serve hot.

Nutritional Information:
- Serving Size: 1/4 of the recipe
- Servings: 4
- Calories per serving: approximately 300
- Total Fat: 20g
- Carbohydrates: 10g Fiber: 2g Protein: 25g

Cooking Time:
- Prep Time: 10 minutes
- Cooking Time: 20 minutes

13. Italian Seafood Risotto

Ingredients:
- 1 cup Arborio rice
- 4 cups seafood broth or chicken broth
- 1/2 cup dry white wine
- 1 shallot, finely chopped
- 2 cloves garlic, minced
- 1 lb mixed seafood (such as shrimp, scallops, mussels, clams)
- 1/4 cup grated Parmesan cheese
- 2 tablespoons unsalted butter
- Salt and pepper to taste
- Chopped fresh parsley for garnish
- Lemon wedges for serving

Instructions:
1. In a saucepan, heat seafood broth over low heat and keep it warm.
2. In a separate large skillet or pot, heat olive oil over medium heat.
3. Add finely chopped shallot and minced garlic to the skillet. Cook until softened, about 2-3 minutes.
4. Add Arborio rice to the skillet and cook, stirring constantly, for 1-2 minutes until the rice is translucent around the edges.
5. Pour in dry white wine and cook, stirring frequently, until the wine is absorbed.
6. Add a ladleful of warm seafood broth to the rice and cook, stirring frequently, until the broth is absorbed.
7. Continue adding ladlefuls of warm broth to the rice, stirring frequently, and allowing each addition to be absorbed before adding more. Cook until the rice is creamy and tender, about 18-20 minutes.
8. In the last 5 minutes of cooking, stir in mixed seafood and cook until the seafood is cooked through.
9. Stir in grated Parmesan cheese and unsalted butter until melted and creamy.
10. Season with salt and pepper to taste.
11. Remove from heat and let the risotto rest for a few minutes.
12. Garnish with chopped fresh parsley and serve hot with lemon wedges.

Nutritional Information:
- Serving Size: 1/4 of the recipe
- Servings: 4
- Calories per serving: approximately 350
- Total Fat: 10g
- Carbohydrates: 40g
- Fiber: 2g
- Protein: 20g

Cooking Time:
- Prep Time: 10 minutes
- Cooking Time: 30 minutes

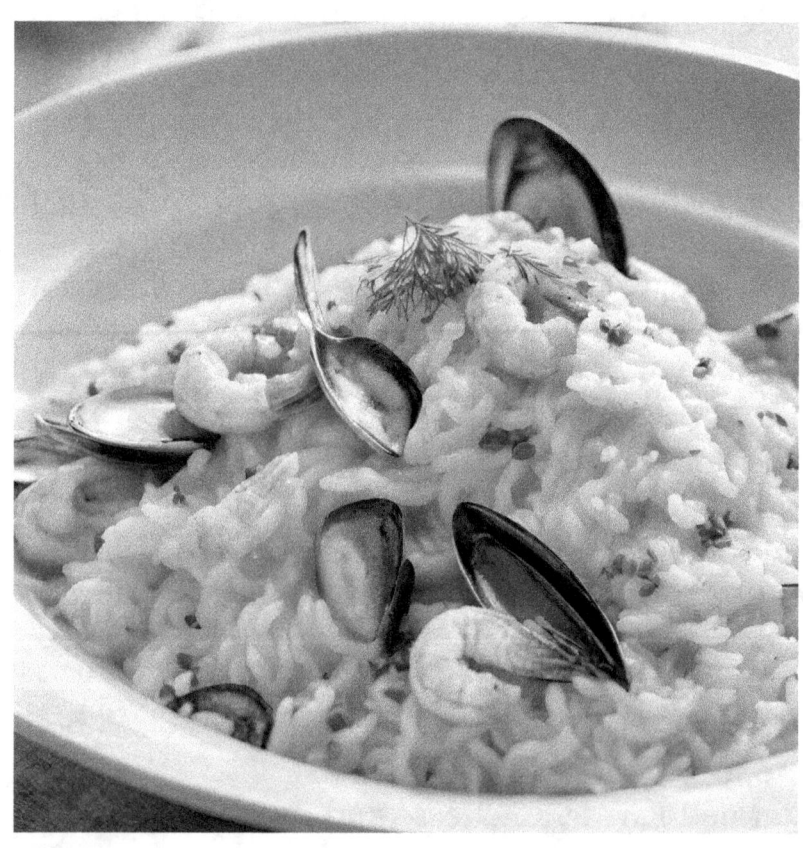

14. Vietnamese Shrimp Summer Rolls

Ingredients:
- 12 rice paper wrappers
- 1 lb shrimp, peeled, deveined, and cooked
- 2 cups vermicelli rice noodles, cooked
- 1 cup shredded lettuce
- 1 cucumber, julienned
- 1 carrot, julienned
- 1/4 cup fresh mint leaves
- 1/4 cup fresh cilantro leaves
- 1/4 cup fresh basil leaves
- Hoisin sauce for dipping
- Peanut sauce for dipping

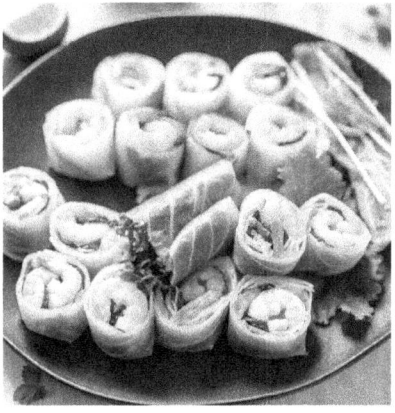

Instructions:
1. Fill a shallow dish with warm water.
2. Dip one rice paper wrapper into the warm water for a few seconds until it softens.
3. Place the softened rice paper wrapper on a clean, damp kitchen towel.
4. Arrange cooked shrimp, vermicelli rice noodles, shredded lettuce, julienned cucumber, julienned carrot, fresh mint leaves, fresh cilantro leaves, and fresh basil leaves on the bottom third of the rice paper wrapper.
5. Fold the bottom of the rice paper wrapper over the filling, then fold in the sides, and roll tightly to enclose the filling.
6. Repeat with the remaining rice paper wrappers and filling ingredients.
7. Serve the Vietnamese shrimp summer rolls with hoisin sauce and peanut sauce for dipping.

Nutritional Information:
- Serving Size: 1 roll
- Servings: 12
- Calories per serving: approximately 100
- Total Fat: 1g
- Carbohydrates: 20g
- Fiber: 1g Protein: 5g

Cooking Time:
- Prep Time: 20 minutes
- Cooking Time: 10 minutes (for cooking noodles and shrimp)

15. Greek Grilled Swordfish

Ingredients:
- 4 swordfish steaks
- 1/4 cup olive oil
- Zest and juice of 1 lemon
- 2 cloves garlic, minced
- 1 tablespoon chopped fresh oregano
- 1 tablespoon chopped fresh parsley
- Salt and pepper to taste
- Lemon wedges for serving

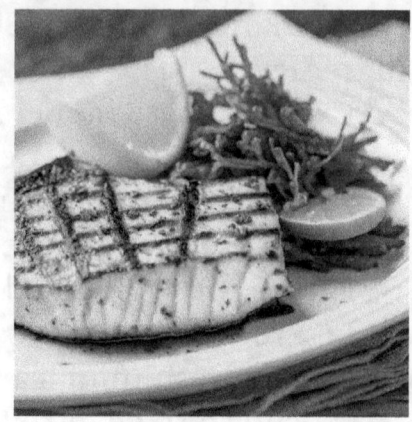

Instructions:
1. In a bowl, whisk together olive oil, lemon zest, lemon juice, minced garlic, chopped oregano, chopped parsley, salt, and pepper to make the marinade.
2. Place swordfish steaks in a shallow dish and pour the marinade over them. Marinate for at least 30 minutes to 1 hour.
3. Preheat grill to medium-high heat.
4. Remove swordfish steaks from the marinade and shake off any excess.
5. Grill the swordfish steaks for 4-5 minutes per side, or until they are cooked through and have grill marks.
6. Remove from the grill and let them rest for a few minutes.
7. Serve the Greek grilled swordfish hot with lemon wedges.

Nutritional Information:
- Serving Size: 1 swordfish steak
- Servings: 4
- Calories per serving: approximately 250
- Total Fat: 10g
- Carbohydrates: 0g
- Fiber: 0g
- Protein: 35g

Cooking Time:
- Prep Time: 10 minutes (plus marinating time)
- Cooking Time: 10 minutes

16. Japanese Teriyaki Glazed Salmon

Ingredients:

- 4 salmon fillets
- 1/4 cup soy sauce
- 2 tablespoons mirin
- 2 tablespoons sake (optional)
- 2 tablespoons brown sugar
- 1 tablespoon honey
- 2 cloves garlic, minced
- 1 teaspoon grated ginger
- Sesame seeds for garnish
- Sliced green onions for garnish

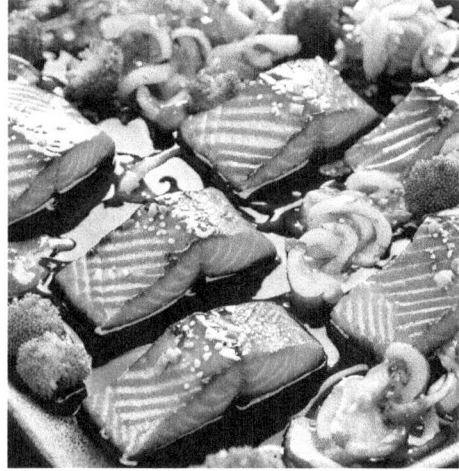

Instructions:

1. In a bowl, whisk together soy sauce, mirin, sake (if using), brown sugar, honey, minced garlic, and grated ginger to make the teriyaki sauce.
2. Place salmon fillets in a shallow dish and pour the teriyaki sauce over them. Marinate for at least 30 minutes, up to 2 hours.
3. Preheat grill to medium-high heat.
4. Remove salmon fillets from the marinade and shake off excess marinade.
5. Grill the salmon fillets for 4-5 minutes per side, or until the fish flakes easily with a fork and is cooked through.
6. Remove from the grill and let them rest for a few minutes.
7. Garnish with sesame seeds and sliced green onions.
8. Serve the Japanese teriyaki glazed salmon hot.

Nutritional Information:

- Serving Size: 1 salmon fillet
- Servings: 4
- Calories per serving: approximately 250
- Total Fat: 10g
- Carbohydrates: 10g
- Fiber: 0g
- Protein: 30g

Cooking Time:

- Prep Time: 10 minutes (plus marinating time)
- Cooking Time: 10 minutes

17. American New England Clam Chowder

Ingredients:
- 2 tablespoons unsalted butter
- 1 onion, chopped
- 2 stalks celery, chopped
- 2 cloves garlic, minced
- 3 cups diced potatoes
- 2 cups clam juice
- 2 cups chicken broth
- 2 cups chopped clams, with juice
- 2 cups half-and-half
- 2 tablespoons all-purpose flour
- Salt and pepper to taste
- Chopped fresh parsley for garnish
- Oyster crackers for serving

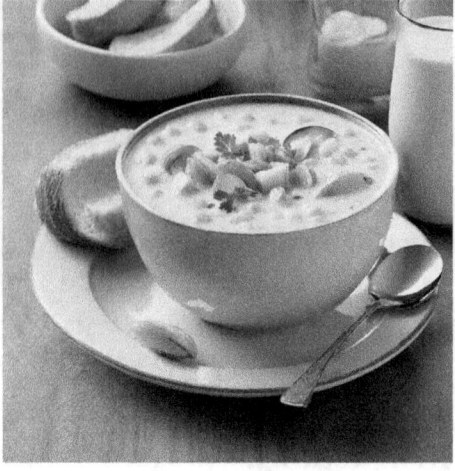

Instructions:
1. In a large pot, melt unsalted butter over medium heat.
2. Add chopped onion, chopped celery, and minced garlic to the pot. Cook until softened, about 5-7 minutes.
3. Stir in diced potatoes, clam juice, and chicken broth. Bring to a simmer and cook until the potatoes are tender, about 15 minutes.
4. In a small bowl, whisk together half-and-half and all-purpose flour until smooth. Pour into the pot and stir to combine.
5. Add chopped clams with their juice to the pot. Cook for an additional 5 minutes until heated through.
6. Season with salt and pepper to taste.
7. Ladle the New England clam chowder into bowls and garnish with chopped fresh parsley.
8. Serve hot with oyster crackers on the side.

Nutritional Information:
- Serving Size: 1/4 of the recipe
- Servings: 4
- Calories per serving: approximately 350
- Total Fat: 15g
- Carbohydrates: 35g Fiber: 3g Protein: 20g

Cooking Time:
- Prep Time: 15 minutes
- Cooking Time: 30 minutes

18. Spanish Seafood Paella

Ingredients:
- 1 lb mixed seafood (such as shrimp, mussels, clams, squid), cleaned and deveined
- 2 tablespoons olive oil
- 1 onion, chopped
- 3 cloves garlic, minced
- 1 red bell pepper, diced
- 1 tomato, diced
- 1 1/2 cups Arborio rice
- 3 cups chicken broth
- 1 teaspoon smoked paprika
- 1 teaspoon saffron threads
- Salt and pepper to taste
- Lemon wedges for serving
- Chopped fresh parsley for garnish

Instructions:
1. Preheat oven to 375°F (190°C).
2. Heat olive oil in a large oven-safe skillet or paella pan over medium heat.
3. Add chopped onion, minced garlic, diced red bell pepper, and diced tomato to the skillet. Cook until softened, about 5-7 minutes.
4. Stir in Arborio rice, smoked paprika, and saffron threads. Cook for 2-3 minutes until the rice is coated with oil.
5. Pour in chicken broth and bring to a simmer. Cook for 10-12 minutes, stirring occasionally, until the rice is partially cooked and most of the liquid is absorbed.
6. Nestle cleaned and deveined seafood into the rice mixture.
7. Transfer the skillet to the preheated oven and bake for 15-20 minutes, or until the seafood is cooked through and the rice is tender.
8. Remove from the oven and let it rest for a few minutes.
9. Season with salt and pepper to taste.
10. Garnish with chopped fresh parsley and serve hot with lemon wedges.

Nutritional Information
- Calories per serving: approximately 400
- Total Fat: 10g
- Fiber: 2g
- Protein: 25g

Cooking Time:
- Prep Time: 20 minutes
- Cooking Time: 45 minutes

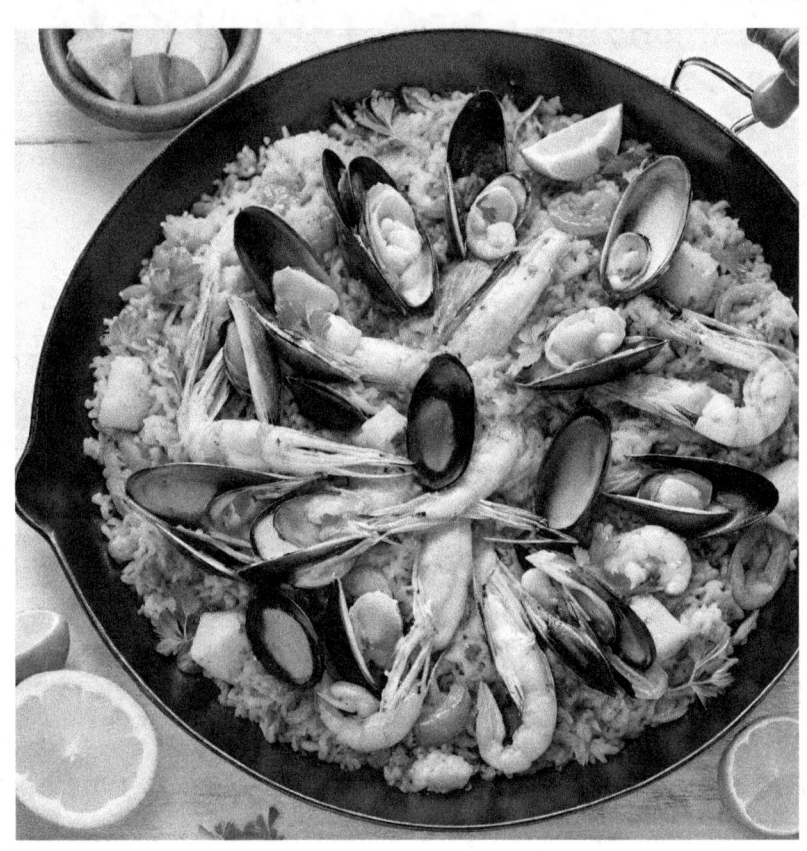

19. Thai Spicy Basil Squid (Pad Kra Pao Pla Meuk)

Ingredients:
- 1 lb squid, cleaned and sliced into rings
- 2 tablespoons vegetable oil
- 4 cloves garlic, minced
- 2 Thai bird's eye chilies, thinly sliced
- 1 bell pepper, sliced
- 1 onion, sliced
- 1 cup fresh basil leaves
- 2 tablespoons oyster sauce
- 1 tablespoon soy sauce
- 1 tablespoon fish sauce
- 1 teaspoon sugar
- Lime wedges for serving
- Cooked rice for serving

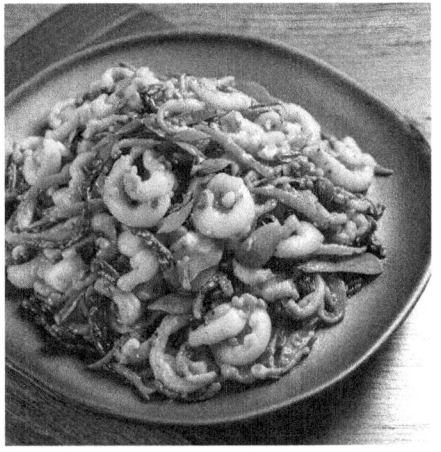

Instructions:
1. Heat vegetable oil in a wok or large skillet over high heat.
2. Add minced garlic and sliced Thai bird's eye chilies to the wok. Stir-fry for 30 seconds until fragrant.
3. Add sliced bell pepper and onion to the wok. Stir-fry for 2-3 minutes until slightly softened.
4. Add cleaned and sliced squid to the wok. Stir-fry for 2-3 minutes until the squid is cooked through.
5. Stir in oyster sauce, soy sauce, fish sauce, and sugar. Cook for another minute until well combined.
6. Add fresh basil leaves to the wok and toss to wilt.
7. Remove from heat and serve the Thai spicy basil squid hot with lime wedges and cooked rice.

Nutritional Information:
- Serving Size: 1/4 of the recipe
- Servings: 4
- Calories per serving: approximately 200
- Total Fat: 6g
- Carbohydrates: 10g
- Fiber: 2g
- Protein: 25g

Cooking Time:
- Prep Time: 15 minutes
- Cooking Time: 10 minutes

20. Italian Linguine with Clams

Ingredients:
- 12 oz linguine
- 2 tablespoons olive oil
- 4 cloves garlic, minced
- 1/4 teaspoon red pepper flakes
- 1/2 cup dry white wine
- 2 dozen littleneck clams, scrubbed
- 1/4 cup chopped fresh parsley
- Salt and pepper to taste
- Lemon wedges for serving

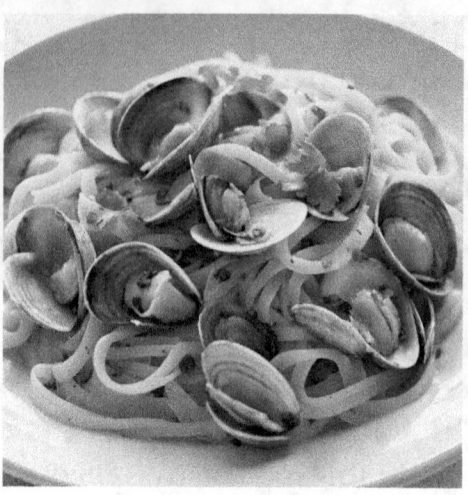

Instructions:
1. Cook linguine according to package instructions until al dente. Drain and set aside.
2. In a large skillet, heat olive oil over medium heat.
3. Add minced garlic and red pepper flakes to the skillet. Cook for 1 minute until fragrant.
4. Pour in dry white wine and bring to a simmer.
5. Add scrubbed littleneck clams to the skillet. Cover and cook for 5-7 minutes until the clams have opened.
6. Discard any unopened clams.
7. Stir in chopped fresh parsley and cooked linguine. Toss to combine.
8. Season with salt and pepper to taste.
9. Serve the Italian linguine with clams hot with lemon wedges.

Nutritional Information:
- Serving Size: 1/4 of the recipe
- Servings: 4
- Calories per serving: approximately 300
- Total Fat: 6g
- Carbohydrates: 45g
- Fiber: 2g
- Protein: 15g

Cooking Time:
- Prep Time: 10 minutes
- Cooking Time: 20 minutes

21. French Bouillabaisse

Ingredients:
- 1 lb mixed seafood (such as fish fillets, shrimp, mussels, clams)
- 2 tablespoons olive oil
- 1 onion, chopped
- 2 cloves garlic, minced
- 1 fennel bulb, sliced
- 1 carrot, sliced
- 1 stalk celery, sliced
- 1/2 cup dry white wine
- 1 can (14 oz) diced tomatoes
- 4 cups fish broth or seafood broth
- 1 bay leaf
- 1 teaspoon dried thyme
- Salt and pepper to taste
- Saffron threads for garnish
- Chopped fresh parsley for garnish
- Toasted bread for serving

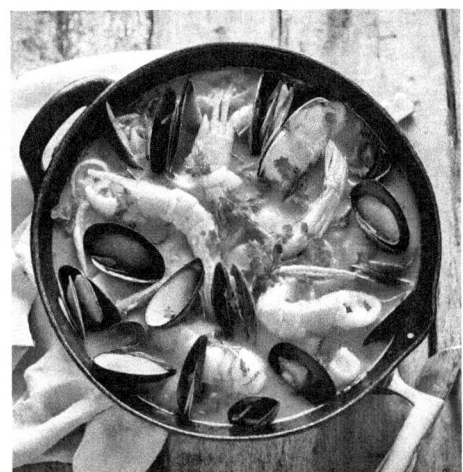

Instructions:
1. Heat olive oil in a large pot over medium heat.
2. Add chopped onion, minced garlic, sliced fennel bulb, sliced carrot, and sliced celery to the pot. Cook until softened, about 5-7 minutes.
3. Pour in dry white wine and simmer for 2-3 minutes until slightly reduced.
4. Add diced tomatoes, fish broth or seafood broth, bay leaf, and dried thyme to the pot. Bring to a boil, then reduce heat to low and let it simmer for 15-20 minutes.
5. Season with salt and pepper to taste.
6. Add mixed seafood to the pot and cook for 5-7 minutes until the seafood is cooked through.
7. Remove from heat and discard the bay leaf.
8. Ladle the French bouillabaisse into bowls.
9. Garnish with saffron threads and chopped fresh parsley.
10. Serve hot with toasted bread.

Nutritional Information: Serving Size: 1/4 of the recipe Servings: 4
- Calories per serving: approximately 300
- Total Fat: 10g Carbohydrates: 15g Fiber: 4g Protein: 30g

Cooking Time: 40 minutes

22. Thai Coconut Curry Shrimp

Ingredients:
- 1 lb shrimp, peeled and deveined
- 2 tablespoons red curry paste
- 1 can (14 oz) coconut milk
- 1 red bell pepper, sliced
- 1 yellow bell pepper, sliced
- 1 onion, sliced
- 1 zucchini, sliced
- 1 cup snap peas
- 2 tablespoons fish sauce
- 1 tablespoon brown sugar
- Juice of 1 lime
- Fresh cilantro for garnish
- Cooked rice for serving

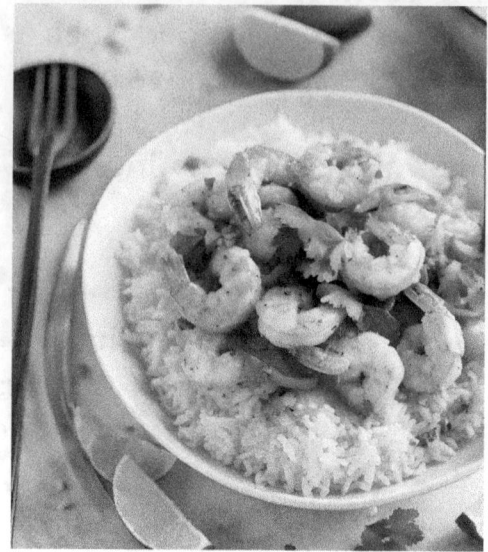

Instructions:
1. In a large skillet or wok, heat coconut milk over medium heat.
2. Add red curry paste to the skillet and stir to combine.
3. Add sliced red bell pepper, yellow bell pepper, onion, zucchini, and snap peas to the skillet. Cook for 5-7 minutes until the vegetables are tender.
4. Stir in peeled and deveined shrimp, fish sauce, brown sugar, and lime juice. Cook for an additional 3-4 minutes until the shrimp is pink and cooked through.
5. Remove from heat and garnish with fresh cilantro.
6. Serve the Thai coconut curry shrimp hot with cooked rice.

Nutritional Information:
- Serving Size: 1/4 of the recipe
- Servings: 4
- Calories per serving: approximately 250
- Total Fat: 10g
- Carbohydrates: 15g
- Fiber: 3g
- Protein: 20g

Cooking Time:
- Prep Time: 15 minutes
- Cooking Time: 15 minutes

8-WEEK MEAL PLAN.

Week 1: Introduction to Lymphatic Health

Day 1:
- **Breakfast:** Green Smoothie (Spinach, Green Apple, Lemon, Ginger, and Flaxseed)
- **Lunch:** Quinoa Salad with Mixed Vegetables and Lemon-Tahini Dressing
- **Dinner:** Baked Salmon with Steamed Broccoli and Brown Rice

Day 2:
- **Breakfast:** Overnight Oats with Almond Milk, Chia Seeds, and Berries
- **Lunch:** Avocado and Turkey Breast Wrap with Whole Grain Tortilla
- **Dinner:** Lentil Soup with Carrots, Celery, and Kale

Day 3:
- **Breakfast:** Fruit Salad with a Drizzle of Lemon Juice and a Sprinkle of Pumpkin Seeds
- **Lunch:** Chickpea and Cucumber Salad with Olive Oil and Herb Dressing
- **Dinner:** Grilled Chicken Breast with Quinoa and Roasted Asparagus

Day 4:
- **Breakfast:** Smoothie Bowl with Spinach, Banana, Almond Milk, Topped with Granola
- **Lunch:** Sardine Salad on Whole Grain Bread with Avocado
- **Dinner:** Turkey Meatballs in Tomato Sauce with Zucchini Noodles

Day 5:
- **Breakfast:** Scrambled Eggs with Spinach and Mushrooms
- **Lunch:** Sweet Potato and Black Bean Buddha Bowl
- **Dinner:** Grilled Tilapia with Mixed Greens Salad

Day 6:
- **Breakfast:** Chia Pudding with Coconut Milk and Mixed Berries
- **Lunch:** Chicken Caesar Salad with Homemade Dressing
- **Dinner:** Vegetable Stir-fry with Tofu and Brown Rice

Day 7:
- **Breakfast:** Avocado Toast on Whole Grain Bread with Hemp Seeds
- **Lunch:** Quinoa Tabbouleh
- **Dinner:** Baked Cod with Steamed Green Beans and Almonds

Week 2: Diversifying Your Palette
Day 1:
- **Breakfast:** Pear and Walnut Oatmeal (Steel-cut oats, diced pear, crushed walnuts, cinnamon)
- **Lunch:** Roasted Beet and Goat Cheese Salad (Mixed greens, roasted beets, goat cheese, walnuts, balsamic vinaigrette)
- **Dinner:** Stuffed Bell Peppers (Quinoa, black beans, corn, tomatoes, avocado topping)

Day 2:
- **Breakfast:** Greek Yogurt with Honey and Mixed Nuts
- **Lunch:** Chicken Avocado Salad (Romaine, grilled chicken, avocado, cucumber, olive oil dressing)
- **Dinner:** Baked Haddock with a side of Sautéed Spinach and Garlic Quinoa

Day 3:
- **Breakfast:** Banana Almond Smoothie (Banana, almond butter, almond milk, spinach)
- **Lunch:** Lentil and Sweet Potato Curry with Brown Rice
- **Dinner:** Roasted Turkey Breast with Brussels Sprouts and Sweet Potato Mash

Day 4:
- **Breakfast:** Spinach and Feta Omelette with Whole Grain Toast
- **Lunch:** Quinoa Stuffed Avocados (Quinoa, tomato, cucumber, lemon juice)
- **Dinner:** Grilled Shrimp over Mixed Greens with a Lemon-Herb Dressing

Day 5:
- **Breakfast:** Blueberry and Almond Butter Toast on Ezekiel Bread
- **Lunch:** Turkey and Cranberry Wrap (Whole grain wrap, turkey breast, cranberry sauce, mixed greens)
- **Dinner:** Lemon Garlic Salmon with Asparagus and a side of Farro

Day 6:
- **Breakfast:** Carrot and Ginger Juice with a side of Whole Grain Toast and Avocado
- **Lunch:** Caprese Salad with Balsamic Glaze (Tomato, mozzarella, basil)
- **Dinner:** Chicken Stir-Fry with Broccoli, Bell Pepper, and Cashews on Brown Rice

Day 7:
- **Breakfast:** Chia and Berry Parfait (Chia seeds, coconut milk, mixed berries, granola)
- **Lunch:** Spinach and Quinoa Salad with Lemon Vinaigrette
- **Dinner:** Baked Eggplant Parmesan with a Side Salad

Week 3: Mastering Mindful Eating

Day 1:
- **Breakfast:** Mango and Spinach Smoothie (Mango, spinach, coconut water, lime juice)
- **Lunch:** Zucchini Noodles with Avocado Pesto and Cherry Tomatoes
- **Dinner:** Moroccan Spiced Chickpea Stew with Couscous

Day 2:
- **Breakfast:** Poached Eggs on Avocado Toast with a sprinkle of Chili Flakes
- **Lunch:** Mediterranean Tuna Salad (Tuna, mixed greens, olives, feta, cucumber)
- **Dinner:** Ginger Soy Glazed Salmon with Steamed Bok Choy and Wild Rice

Day 3:
- **Breakfast:** Coconut Milk Yogurt with Granola and Kiwi
- **Lunch:** Roasted Cauliflower Soup with a side of Whole Grain Bread
- **Dinner:** Herb Roasted Chicken Thighs with Roasted Root Vegetables

Day 4:
- **Breakfast:** Apple Cinnamon Quinoa Breakfast Bowl
- **Lunch:** Kale Caesar Salad with Grilled Chicken and Homemade Caesar Dressing
- **Dinner:** Vegetarian Chili with Avocado and Whole Grain Tortilla Chips

Day 5:
- **Breakfast:** Green Tea Smoothie (Green tea, banana, almond milk, honey)
- **Lunch:** Soba Noodle Salad with Peanut Dressing (Soba noodles, bell pepper, carrot, cilantro)
- **Dinner:** Grilled Portobello Mushrooms with Quinoa Salad

Day 6:
- **Breakfast:** Baked Sweet Potato with Almond Butter and Banana Slices
- **Lunch:** Cold Lentil Salad with Cucumbers, Tomatoes, and Feta Cheese
- **Dinner:** Cauliflower Steak with Green Beans and a Side of Mashed Potatoes

Day 7:
- **Breakfast:** Avocado and Egg Breakfast Bowl (Quinoa, spinach, poached egg, avocado)
- **Lunch:** Smoked Salmon and Avocado Wrap with Whole Grain Tortilla
- **Dinner:** Ratatouille with Baked Chicken Breast

Week 4: Exploring New Flavors

Day 1:
- **Breakfast:** Kiwi and Strawberry Smoothie Bowl with Chia Seeds
- **Lunch:** Asian Cabbage Salad with Sesame Ginger Dressing
- **Dinner:** Garlic Lemon Chicken with Cauliflower Rice and Steamed Green Beans

Day 2:
- **Breakfast:** Avocado and Egg on Rye Bread with Crushed Red Pepper
- **Lunch:** Butternut Squash Soup with a side of Arugula Salad
- **Dinner:** Grilled Mahi-Mahi with Mango Salsa and Wild Rice

Day 3:
- **Breakfast:** Oatmeal with Coconut Milk, Pear, and Walnuts
- **Lunch:** Mediterranean Quinoa Bowl with Hummus and Grilled Vegetables
- **Dinner:** Beef Stir-Fry with Broccoli and Brown Rice

Day 4:
- **Breakfast:** Pumpkin Spice Smoothie (Pumpkin puree, banana, almond milk, pumpkin spice)
- **Lunch:** Spinach and Goat Cheese Stuffed Portobello Mushrooms
- **Dinner:** Baked Cod with a Pistachio Crust and Roasted Brussels Sprouts

Day 5:
- **Breakfast:** Cottage Cheese with Pineapple Chunks and Flaxseed
- **Lunch:** Turkey and Spinach Salad with Cranberries and Almonds
- **Dinner:** Spaghetti Squash with Tomato Basil Sauce and Grilled Chicken Strips

Day 6:
- **Breakfast:** Banana and Almond Milk Smoothie with a Dash of Cinnamon
- **Lunch:** Cucumber and Avocado Sushi Rolls with Tamari Sauce
- **Dinner:** Lemon Herb Roasted Chicken with Quinoa and Steamed Carrots

Day 7:
- **Breakfast:** Scrambled Tofu with Spinach and Tomatoes on Whole Grain Toast
- **Lunch:** Carrot and Ginger Salad with Grilled Shrimp
- **Dinner:** Vegetarian Paella with Bell Peppers, Peas, and Artichokes

Week 5: Honoring Seasonal Ingredients

Day 1:
- **Breakfast:** Apple Cider Vinegar Tonic and a Warm Bowl of Oatmeal with Fresh Berries
- **Lunch:** Kale and Apple Salad with Pecans and Dijon Vinaigrette
- **Dinner:** Roasted Chicken with Butternut Squash and Cranberries

Day 2:
- **Breakfast:** Green Juice (Kale, Apple, Lemon, Ginger) and Whole Grain Toast with Avocado
- **Lunch:** Roasted Beet and Carrot Salad with Quinoa
- **Dinner:** Grilled Salmon with Asparagus and Wild Rice Pilaf

Day 3:
- **Breakfast:** Buckwheat Pancakes with Maple Syrup and Fresh Berries
- **Lunch:** Broccoli and Almond Soup with a Side of Rye Bread
- **Dinner:** Turkey Meatloaf with Mashed Sweet Potatoes and Green Beans

Day 4:
- **Breakfast:** Chia Seed Pudding with Seasonal Fruits
- **Lunch:** Spinach and Feta Quiche with a Mixed Greens Salad
- **Dinner:** Baked Trout with Lemon Dill Sauce, Brown Rice, and Steamed Zucchini

Day 5:
- **Breakfast:** Pear and Walnut Salad with Yogurt
- **Lunch:** Avocado Chicken Salad Wrapped in Collard Greens
- **Dinner:** Eggplant and Chickpea Stew with Couscous

Day 6:
- **Breakfast:** Matcha Green Tea Smoothie with Banana and Spinach
- **Lunch:** Sweet Potato and Black Bean Chili
- **Dinner:** Quinoa Stuffed Bell Peppers with a Side of Steamed Broccoli

Day 7:
- **Breakfast:** Mixed Berry and Almond Milk Smoothie
- **Lunch:** Zucchini Noodle Salad with Peanut Sauce
- **Dinner:** Grilled Portobello Mushrooms with Quinoa Salad and Steamed Peas

Week 6:

Day 1:
- **Breakfast:** Raspberry and Kiwi Parfait with Granola
- **Lunch:** Lentil Tabouleh with Cucumber and Tomato
- **Dinner:** Rosemary Lemon Chicken with Roasted Sweet Potatoes and Green Beans

Day 2:
- **Breakfast:** Toasted Whole Grain Bread with Avocado and Tomato Slices
- **Lunch:** Cold Quinoa Salad with Mango and Cilantro
- **Dinner:** Seared Scallops with Cauliflower Mash and Sautéed Kale

Day 3:
- **Breakfast:** Smoothie with Peach, Banana, and Oat Milk
- **Lunch:** Vegan Taco Salad with Walnut Meat and Avocado Lime Dressing
- **Dinner:** Balsamic Glazed Steak Rolls with Vegetables and Side Salad

Day 4:
- **Breakfast:** Poached Pear with Cinnamon and Honey over Cottage Cheese
- **Lunch:** Rainbow Vegetable Spring Rolls with Peanut Dipping Sauce
- **Dinner:** Moroccan Lentil Soup with Whole Grain Bread

Day 5:
- **Breakfast:** Blueberry Muffins made with Almond Flour
- **Lunch:** Grilled Peach and Chicken Salad with Balsamic Reduction
- **Dinner:** Shrimp and Asparagus Stir Fry over Quinoa

Day 6:
- **Breakfast:** Avocado, Spinach, and Egg Breakfast Sandwich on Whole Grain Bagel
- **Lunch:** Butternut Squash and Arugula Wrap
- **Dinner:** Lemon Garlic Tilapia with Roasted Parsnips and a Spinach Salad

Day 7:
- **Breakfast:** Overnight Oats with Coconut Milk, Mango, and Pistachios
- **Lunch:** Sardine Salad on Whole Grain Crackers with a Side of Sliced Cucumbers
- **Dinner:** Vegetarian Mushroom Stroganoff with a Side of Roasted Brussels Sprouts

Week 7:

Day 1:
- **Breakfast:** Mexican-style scrambled eggs with avocado and tomato salsa
- **Lunch:** Greek salad with chickpeas, olives, cucumber, tomato, feta, and a lemon-olive oil dressing
- **Dinner:** Indian lentil dal with turmeric rice and steamed green beans

Day 2:
- **Breakfast:** French whole grain toast with smashed avocado and radish slices
- **Lunch:** Japanese sushi bowl with brown rice, avocado, cucumber, carrot, and a side of miso soup
- **Dinner:** Moroccan chicken tagine with apricots, olives, and couscous

Day 3:
- **Breakfast:** Spanish omelette with potatoes and onions, served with a side of mixed greens
- **Lunch:** Italian caprese sandwich with tomato, mozzarella, basil on whole grain bread
- **Dinner:** Thai green curry with tofu, broccoli, bell pepper, and brown rice

Day 4:
- **Breakfast:** German apple pancake with cinnamon and a side of yogurt
- **Lunch:** Lebanese tabbouleh with parsley, tomato, mint, quinoa, and a lemon dressing
- **Dinner:** Cuban black beans and rice with a side of avocado and salsa

Day 5:
- **Breakfast:** Swedish oat porridge with lingonberries and almonds
- **Lunch:** Ethiopian lentil stew with injera (substitute with whole grain flatbread if needed)
- **Dinner:** Korean bibimbap with mixed vegetables, a fried egg, and brown rice, served with gochujang sauce

Day 6:
- **Breakfast:** English breakfast tea with whole grain scones, clotted cream, and strawberries
- **Lunch:** Mediterranean falafel wrap with tahini sauce, lettuce, and tomato
- **Dinner:** Italian vegetable minestrone soup with a side of whole grain garlic bread

Day 7:
- **Breakfast:** Dutch baby pancake with blueberries and a dusting of powdered sugar
- **Lunch:** Russian beet salad with walnuts, prunes, and a side of whole grain crackers
- **Dinner:** Brazilian fish stew (moqueca) with bell peppers, tomatoes, and lime, served over quinoa

Week 8:
Day 1:
- **Breakfast:** Baked oatmeal with apples, cinnamon, and nutmeg
- **Lunch:** Warm butternut squash and kale salad with cranberries and pecans
- **Dinner:** Roast chicken with root vegetables and a side of wild rice

Day 2:
- **Breakfast:** Pumpkin spice smoothie with banana, pumpkin puree, almond milk, and a touch of maple syrup
- **Lunch:** Roasted vegetable wrap with hummus in a whole grain tortilla
- **Dinner:** Beef and vegetable stew with a side of crusty whole grain bread

Day 3:
- **Breakfast:** Pear and ginger compote over Greek yogurt with a sprinkle of granola
- **Lunch:** Spicy sweet potato soup with a swirl of coconut milk and a side of whole grain toast
- **Dinner:** Baked salmon with dill, lemon, and steamed asparagus

Day 4:
- **Breakfast:** Savory mushroom and spinach crepes
- **Lunch:** Quinoa and black bean stuffed acorn squash
- **Dinner:** Turkey meatballs in tomato sauce with spaghetti squash

Day 5:
- **Breakfast:** Caramelized banana and walnut oatmeal
- **Lunch:** Chicken and avocado salad with a mustard vinaigrette
- **Dinner:** Vegetarian chili with a side of cornbread (use whole grain flour)

Day 6:
- **Breakfast:** Zucchini bread made with almond flour and honey
- **Lunch:** Hearty lentil and vegetable soup
- **Dinner:** Grilled portobello mushrooms with herb quinoa salad

Day 7:
- **Breakfast:** Apple cinnamon quinoa breakfast bowl
- **Lunch:** Roasted beet and goat cheese arugula salad
- **Dinner:** Stuffed bell peppers with ground turkey, quinoa, tomatoes, and spices

FOOD TRACKER JORNAL

	BREAKFAST	LUNCH	DINNER	SNACKS &
MON				
				WATER
TUE				
				WATER
WED				
				WATER
THU				
				WATER
FRI				**FOODS TO AVOID**
SAT				
SUN				

What does a typical day of eating look like for you? Include all meals, snacks, and beverages.

FOOD TRACKER JORNAL

	BREAKFAST	LUNCH	DINNER	SNACKS &
MON				WATER
TUE				WATER
WED				WATER
THU				WATER
FRI				**FOODS TO AVOID**
SAT				
SUN				

What are your main reasons for wanting to follow a lymphatic diet? Are you seeking to improve your overall health, address specific health issues, or both?

....

....

....

....

....

....

....

....

What do you anticipate will be your biggest challenges in adopting a lymphatic diet? Consider food preferences, lifestyle, and any social or emotional obstacles.?

....

....

....

....

....

FOOD TRACKER JORNAL

	BREAKFAST	LUNCH	DINNER	SNACKS &
MON				
				WATER
TUE				
				WATER
WED				
				WATER
THU				
				WATER
FRI				**FOODS TO AVOID**
SAT				
SUN				

What specific health or wellness goals do you hope to achieve by following a lymphatic diet? How will you measure your progress towards these goals?

....

....

....

....

....

....

....

How familiar are you with the lymphatic system and its role in your health? What are you hoping to learn more about?

....

....

....

....

....

FOOD TRACKER JORNAL

	BREAKFAST	LUNCH	DINNER	SNACKS &
MON				WATER
TUE				WATER
WED				WATER
THU				WATER
FRI				**FOODS TO AVOID**
SAT				
SUN				

How does your current level of physical activity support your lymphatic health? Are there changes you plan to make to become more active?

....

....

....

....

....

Before starting the lymphatic diet, record any symptoms or health issues you are currently experiencing. How might you monitor changes in these symptoms as you progress?

....

....

....

....

....

....

....

....

FOOD TRACKER JORNAL

	BREAKFAST	LUNCH	DINNER	SNACKS &
MON				WATER
TUE				WATER
WED				WATER
THU				WATER
FRI				**FOODS TO AVOID**
SAT				
SUN				

Who in your life can offer you support as you transition to a lymphatic diet? How will you engage them in your journey?

....

....

....

....

....

Are there any supplements you are considering to complement your lymphatic diet? How will you decide which ones might be beneficial for you?

....

....

....

....

....

....

....

....

FOOD TRACKER JORNAL

	BREAKFAST	LUNCH	DINNER	SNACKS &
MON				WATER
TUE				WATER
WED				WATER
THU				WATER
FRI				**FOODS TO AVOID**
SAT				
SUN				

FOOD TRACKER JORNAL

	BREAKFAST	LUNCH	DINNER	SNACKS &
MON				WATER ☐☐☐☐☐☐☐
TUE				WATER ☐☐☐☐☐☐☐
WED				WATER ☐☐☐☐☐☐☐
THU				WATER ☐☐☐☐☐☐☐
FRI				**FOODS TO AVOID**
SAT				
SUN				

FOOD TRACKER JORNAL

	BREAKFAST	LUNCH	DINNER	SNACKS &
MON				WATER
TUE				WATER
WED				WATER
THU				WATER
FRI				**FOODS TO AVOID**
SAT				
SUN				

# FOOD TRACKER JORNAL

	BREAKFAST	LUNCH	DINNER	SNACKS &
MON				WATER ☐☐☐☐☐☐☐
TUE				WATER ☐☐☐☐☐☐☐
WED				WATER ☐☐☐☐☐☐☐
THU				WATER ☐☐☐☐☐☐☐
FRI				**FOODS TO AVOID**
SAT				
SUN				

FOOD TRACKER JORNAL

	BREAKFAST	LUNCH	DINNER	SNACKS &
MON				WATER
TUE				WATER
WED				WATER
THU				WATER
FRI				**FOODS TO AVOID**
SAT				
SUN				

FOOD TRACKER JORNAL

	BREAKFAST	LUNCH	DINNER	SNACKS &
MON				WATER ☐☐☐☐☐☐
TUE				WATER ☐☐☐☐☐☐
WED				WATER ☐☐☐☐☐☐
THU				WATER ☐☐☐☐☐☐
FRI				**FOODS TO AVOID**
SAT				
SUN				

Scan the QR code below to get a surprise bonus!

If you would love to have a one-on-one consultation session with Dr. Kelly Haaland, kindly reach out to us at kellyhaaland2@gmail.com.

www.ingramcontent.com/pod-product-compliance
Lightning Source LLC
Chambersburg PA
CBHW062106220526
45471CB00010B/3624